Will the Last Physician in America Please Turn Off the Lights?
A Look at America s Looming Doctor Shortage

First Printing — September 2004
Second Printing — June 2005
Third Printing — January 2006

ISBN: 0-9759956-0-X

Printed in the United States of America

Practice Support Resources, Inc., Publisher
Additional copies of this book may be ordered by
calling 1-800-967-7790 or online at www.practicesupport.com.

This book is for informational purposes only. It is not intended to constitute legal or
financial advice. If legal, financial, or other professional advice is required, the services
of a competent professional should be sought.

Praise For This Book

"The new Merritt, Hawkins book is light and readable but densely packed with information – a sobering exposition of the deepening problem of physician shortages. It will interest health professionals as well as patients and should be **required reading** for policy makers and politicians who delivered the physician shortage that we are now experiencing and will have to work America out of it."

Richard Cooper, M.D., Health Policy Director, Medical College of Wisconsin

"Anyone who cares about the quality of healthcare in America **has to read this book.** It will both shock and educate you about the critical, skilled people problems that are about to descend upon the robust healthcare scene. Everyone knows about the nursing shortage but in a very few short years there will be a shortage of over 200,000 physicians in this country. As a consequence, waiting times will increase and consumer choice will be limited. It will threaten the very fabric of American healthcare and along the way probably affect the very quality of life we enjoy in the good old USA. **This is a must read!**"

Charles Lauer, Publisher, *Modern Healthcare*

"A timely and **important wake-up call** for anyone interested in health care delivery in America. The book raises serious questions for which we need to find serious answers."

Vicki Pascasio, President & CEO, HealthShare/Texas Hospital Association

Will The Last Physician In America Please Turn Off The Lights?

A Look at America's Looming Doctor Shortage

By James Merritt, Joseph Hawkins, and Phillip B. Miller

The MHA Group
5001 Statesman Drive
Irving, Texas 75063
800-876-0500
469-524-1400
www.mhagroup.com

Acknowledgements

The authors would like to thank Kurt Mosley, Vice President of Business Development for The MHA Group, for his invaluable assistance and expertise in compiling information for this book. We also would like to thank all of our associates at The MHA Group for their exemplary professionalism, camaraderie and commitment.

About the Authors

JAMES MERRITT

James Merritt is President and co-founder of The MHA Group, one of the largest health care staffing and consulting firms in the nation.

Mr. Merritt has over 24 years of health care consulting experience and is a nationally acknowledged health care staffing leader. In 1987, he co-founded Merritt, Hawkins & Associates, the nation's leading permanent placement physician search and consulting firm. Merritt, Hawkins & Associates has since evolved into The MHA Group, an organization of affiliated health care staffing and consulting firms that includes Merritt Hawkins & Associates, Staff Care, Inc., Med Travelers, and RN Demand. Mr. Merritt continues to be actively involved in the daily management of The MHA Group focusing on strategic marketing operations.

Mr. Merritt is widely recognized for his expertise in a broad range of staffing issues, from physician compensation to medical staff planning. Mr. Merritt has consulted with hundreds of hospitals and medical groups regarding physician needs assessment, physician search strategies, compensation, contracts, retention and numerous other related issues. Firms founded or managed by Mr. Merritt have conducted over 30,000 physician search assignments nationwide.

Mr. Merritt has been repeatedly noted for his expertise. His comments have appeared in numerous respected publications, including *The Wall Street Journal, USA Today, Modern Healthcare, Hospitals & Health Networks, American Medical News,* and many others. Mr. Merritt has written dozens of articles on health care staffing issues that have appeared in publications ranging from *Modern Healthcare* to *The Dallas Morning News.*

Mr. Merritt is a frequently requested speaker who has addressed a wide range of health care professional groups throughout the United States and Canada, including the Medical Group Management Association, the Texas Hospital Association and many others.

Mr. Merritt serves on the Board of Directors of Texas Hospital Association/HealthShare and is distinguished as the only member to serve on the Board who is not affiliated with a hospital or other provider of health care services.

Mr. Merritt is originally from Ontario, Canada and now resides in Dallas, Texas.

JOSEPH HAWKINS

Joseph Hawkins is co-founder and Chief Executive Officer of The MHA Group, one of the largest health care staffing and consulting firms in the nation.

Mr. Hawkins has over 24 years of experience in physician search and is considered one of the leading figures in the health care staffing industry. Formerly a divisional vice president with a national physician search firm, Mr. Hawkins co-founded Merritt, Hawkins & Associates, now the nation's largest physician search firm, in 1987. Firms founded or managed by Mr. Hawkins have conducted over 30,000 physician search assignments throughout the United States.

Merritt, Hawkins & Associates is now one of four staffing and consulting firms that comprise The MHA Group, which also includes Staff Care, Inc., Med Travelers, and RN Demand. Mr. Hawkins is responsible for overall strategic operations of The MHA Group's four offices nationwide and its 750 employees.

A pioneer in the field of physician search, Mr. Hawkins helped develop recruiting systems that have been widely imitated throughout the industry. His expertise has been cited in dozens of health care, business and general news publications, including *The Wall Street Journal, Fortune, Modern Healthcare, Hospitals & Health Networks, American Medical News, Medical Economics, Journal of the American Medical Association,* and numerous others.

Mr. Hawkins has written dozens of articles on health care staffing that have appeared in health care and general press outlets ranging from *The Journal of the American Medical Association* to *The Dallas Morning News.*

Mr. Hawkins also has addressed a wide range of health care professional groups across the country on issues ranging from physician compensation to federal physician recruiting guidelines.

A graduate of Florida State University, Mr. Hawkins resides in Dallas, Texas.

PHILLIP B. MILLER

Phillip B. Miller serves as Vice President of Corporate Communications for The MHA Group, the nation's leading health care staffing provider, and has over 18 years of experience in corporate communications and public relations. Mr. Miller has authored or co-authored over 400 articles on issues ranging from physician recruitment, to immigration, to emergency medicine. As a spokesperson for The MHA Group, Mr. Miller has been cited by *The Wall Street Journal, National Public Radio, People* magazine, *The Dallas Morning News* and many other general interest and health care media outlets. Mr. Miller also is the author of the guidebook *L.A.'s 99 Best Hole-in-the-Wall Restaurants*. A graduate of the University of Texas, Austin, Mr. Miller lives in Dallas, Texas.

Contents

Chapter One:
Introduction: The Doctor Won't See You Now

"It's tough to make predictions, especially about the future" -- Yogi Berra

America is running out of physicians, and we hope you will read this book to find out why.

If you would like to skip the fine print, however, you can put our assertion to the test with a simple experiment. Pick up your local Yellow Pages and flip to the physician listings. Find the section that lists the "ologies" – cardiology, dermatology, gastroenterology, or any other "ology" you might prefer.

Call one or more of these offices and ask to set up a new patient appointment. Say you have a chronic problem – though not an emergency – such as back pain or indigestion, or that you need a heart check up or a routine skin exam, as the case may be. The receptionist will ask you about insurance. If you have an insurance plan, and the physician participates in the plan, you'll get an appointment, but it will take you about a month or more to get in.

If you have insurance, but of a kind the physician doesn't accept – and this usually means Medicaid or Medicare – you'll have to try elsewhere. And if you have no insurance at all (and don't have enough money to pay the doctor at the time of your visit), well, you are probably going to have to go the nearest hospital emergency room if you want to see a physician – even if you only have a runny nose or a headache. And even at the ER, you may have no luck accessing the type of physician you need (see Chapter 6.)

How do we know? Because we've already conducted this experiment ourselves. In February and March of 2004, research associates at our company called over 2,500 physicians in 15 major metro markets nationwide. They asked for a new patient appointment. They complained of a variety of non-emergent ailments and asked for the first available appointment. They also asked if the physician accepted Medicaid as a form of payment.

Here's a sample of what we found, focusing on cardiology and obstetrics/gynecology, two of the various medical specialties we researched.

1

Time to a New Physician Appointment / Cardiology*

City, State	Time to Appointment (heart check-up)	Accepts Medicaid
Boston, MA	37 days	11%
Philadelphia, PA	27 days	80%
Portland, OR	25 days	100%
Denver, CO	23 days	20%
New York, NY	22 days	0%
Miami, FL	21 days	40%
Detroit, MI	20 days	65%

Time to a New Physician Appointment / OB/GYN*

City, State	Time to Appointment (annual exam)	Accepts Medicaid
Boston, MA	45 days	56%
Detroit, MI	39 days	40%
San Diego, CA	31 days	80%
Portland, OR	30 days	100%
Philadelphia, PA	28 days	24%
Seattle, WA	26 days	70%
Atlanta, GA	24 days	25%

Source: Merritt, Hawkins & Associates 2004 Survey of Physician Appointment Wait Times

The average wait time for a new patient appointment for the medical specialties we researched typically ranged from two to five weeks. Now, if you think a month or so is a long time to wait for a doctor's appointment, you haven't seen anything yet. Within the next 15 years, the United States will experience a shortage of somewhere between 90,000 to 200,000 physicians. Patients will have to wait three to four months or more to see a physician for non-emergencies, and a routine doctor visit is going to cost two to three times what it does now, whether you are insured or not.

As the chart above suggests, it is medical specialists such as cardiologists who will be the hardest to see. "Primary care" doctors such as family physicians will still be accessible, if not readily available. But in ten to 15 years (and probably right now) the majority of you reading this book won't need to see a family doctor. But you will need to see an orthopedic surgeon for your bum knee, a cardiologist for your blocked arteries, a urologist for your faulty plumbing, an endocrinologist for your obesity related diabetes, or a psychiatrist for the depression brought on by an increasingly angst-ridden society.

When you, or your spouse, or your parents need one, will there be a doctor in the house? Not if things continue as they are. If things continue as they are, the current shortage of nurses, which has driven up hospital errors and patient morbidity, will seem like déjà vu all over again when it comes to doctors.

There is an increasing amount of statistical information available to support this assertion, and some of it is alluded to in this book. Our conclusions also are based on our combined 48 years of experience recruiting doctors, during which time companies we have run have conducted over 30,000 physician recruiting assignments distributed over all 50 states. While we monitor what the academics and the government experts have to say about physician supply and demand, we also live it and breathe it every day from what might be called the "street perspective." We understand how challenging it is to find physicians today, and the difficulties communities face when they are not able to recruit the doctors they need.

Over the past two decades, the challenges posed by physician recruitment have steadily increased. Indeed, at no time in the 24 years that we have been physician recruiters has the process of recruiting physicians been as time and resource-intensive as it is today.

Why are we running short of doctors? Why is it that our best and brightest young people, who once clamored to get into medicine, are now having second thoughts about the profession? Why are many older physicians looking for ways to opt out of patient care? What does the looming physician shortage mean to you and what can be done about it?

For answers to those questions, you *will* have to read the fine print.

Chapter 2:
The Dirty Dozen

Question: What do you call an anesthesiologist just coming out of training?

Answer: "Waiter!"

The joke above, which is a little puzzling today, was considered quite funny in the early to mid-1990s. It was funny because just five or six years ago people thought that medical specialists such as anesthesiologists were going to have a hard time finding work. The idea was that managed care was going to reduce the total number of surgeries performed so dramatically that anesthesiologists would hardly be needed – they would have to resort to waiting tables.

Compare that joke, or the point behind it, to this headline and story that appeared in the May 23, 2003 edition of the *Denver Post:*

"DOCTOR SHORTAGE STALLING SURGERIES"

"Lucrative procedures at cosmetic surgeons' offices and outpatient surgery centers are luring Denver's shrinking pool of anesthesiologists away from urban hospitals."

"The shortage has gotten so bad in the last two months that University of Colorado Hospital has had to shut down operating rooms."

Here are a few other headlines that send a similar message:

"Doctors Vanish From View"
U.S. News & World Report, January 31- Feb. 7, 2005

"Medical Miscalculation Creates Doctor Shortage"
USA Today, March 3, 2005

"Doctor Shortage to Grow Worse"
Kiplinger Forecasts, April 8, 2005

"There's a shortage of specialists. Is anyone listening?"
Academic Medicine, Vol. 77, No. 8/August, 2002

"The coming shortage of physicians in the United States"
New England Journal of Medicine (online version, www.nejm.org) 2/11/2002

"Now forecast is for shortage of physicians"
American Medical News, 1/21/02

"UCLA study reveals there will not be enough surgeons to meet needs of aging population"
UCLA News, July 29, 2003

"Experts predict a shortage of medical specialists to care for future generations"
Knight Ridder Newspapers, Kansas City Star, 12/05/00

"Federal rules create looming physician shortage"
San Jose Mercury News, 11/7/2001

"Doctor shortage looms as threat, professor warns"
Milwaukee Journal Sentinel, 12/9/03

"Federal advisory group predicts physician shortage looming"
American Medical News, 11/3/2003

"Where have all the anesthesiologists gone? Analysis of the national anesthesia worker shortage"
American Society of Anesthesiologists Newsletter, April, 2001

"Neuro Surgeons in short supply"
The Boston Globe, 4/28/04

So how could we have gone from a glut of anesthesiologists and other medical specialists to a shortage in just six or seven years? The quick answer is that *there was no glut.* There have never been too many doctors in America, at least not in the modern age of medicine spanning the last 90 years or so since medical training became the rigorous, regulated process it is today.

After all, have you ever heard of an *unemployed physician?* There aren't any – barring those doctors who are compromised by drug abuse or other questionable behavior.

The problem – or one of them – is that the "experts" perceived there was an overabundance of doctors that was going to culminate in an outright *infestation* if action wasn't taken. That is one reason why we are looking at a serious doctor shortage today. In fact, there are 12 reasons why we are running out of doctors – we call them the **"Dirty Dozen"** – and here they are.

1. The Experts Were Wrong

While you and most other successful and good looking people (we see no harm in flattering our readers) focus on the daily task of making ends meet, there are other people whose job it is to worry about the supply of physicians in America. Some of these people – academics and physicians, mostly – got together in 1980 at the behest of the federal government to report on the national state of physician manpower. This group was called GMENAC – the Graduate Medical Education National Advisory Committee. What GMENAC found was not good. Soon – by the year 2000, in fact – America would have too many physicians – 150,000 too many.

This projection was backed up by subsequent studies, such as the one conducted by the Council on Graduate Medical Education (COGME), the successor to GMENAC. In 1994, COGME projected that there would be 100,000 to 165,000 too many specialist physicians by the year 2000. Supply would outstrip demand by 65%!

An oversupply of specialists was considered bad because many experts believed (and some still do) that the more physicians there are the more health care costs go up. It was considered a good idea to limit the number of specialists to keep health care costs low. Many professional associations and federal bureaucrats embraced this idea. The practical effect was decreased financial support for specialty physician training mandated by the Balanced Budget Act of 1997. The number of residency slots for training specialists such as anesthesiologists and radiologists was reduced and federal spending on residency training was capped.

Moreover, in the last 20 years the number of U.S. medical schools has remained static. The number of medical students graduating each year and the number of residents coming out of U.S. training programs also has remained static, at about 16,000 per year. No one saw a need to increase these numbers – just the opposite, in fact.

In public policy matters of this kind it is always instructive to "follow the money." The federal government is comfortable with the idea that we have too many physicians because physician training is largely funded by taxpayer dollars. The government, through the Medicare program, pays teaching hospitals for each doctor they train – to the aggregate tune of some 11 billion dollars a year. The fewer doctors we need, the less the government has to pay for doctor training. Both federal and state governments also have to foot most of the bill for new or expanded medical schools. That means higher taxes.

How many politicians out there want to call for higher taxes? Just raise your hands.

We thought so.

Major physician organizations such as the American Medical Association (AMA) also have a vested interest in keeping the supply of physicians moderate to low. Fewer physicians mean less competition for existing AMA members, keeping incomes high.

There is good news, however, which is that the experts have come around to our way of thinking – "our" being all the physician recruiters and hospital administrators out there who have been trying to find doctors over the last several years and know how hard it has become.

COGME now endorses a study indicating that the U.S. faces not a surplus of physicians, but a shortage of up to 96,000 doctors by the year 2020. Other respected observers see the potential deficit as being considerably higher. Richard Cooper, MD, of the Wisconsin Medical College, authored a study published in the February, 2002 edition of *Health Affairs,* that projects a shortage of 200,000 doctors by the year 2020.

Here are Dr. Cooper's projections:

	1929	*2000*	*2010*	*2020*
Total Physicians	144,000	772,000	887,300	964,700
Physicians per 100,000 pop.	119	270	283	280
Population in millions	121	286	325	335
Shortage of physicians	N/A	N/A	50,000	200,000

Cooper, et al. *Health Affairs,* Feb. 2002

Even the AMA, which has been a staunch supporter of the surplus point of view, has changed its position. In December, 2003, the AMA's Education committee accepted the idea that physician shortages exist and that a panel be created to research the issue.

Most of the leading academic experts who track physician supply met in Washington, D.C. in May of 2005 at an annual meeting sponsored by the Association of American Medical Colleges (AAMC.) At this meeting, which one of the authors of this book attended, it was generally agreed that previous predictions of a physician surplus had been in error and that steps must be taken to further study and address the challenge presented by the physician shortage.

The AAMC now has taken the position that the number of medical school graduates should be increased by 3,000 per year by the year 2015. However, even this ambitious increase will have a negligible effect on the physician shortage. Consider the following projection, which Edward Salsberg, Director of the AAMC's Center for Workforce Studies made during the Washington, D.C. conference referenced above.

Impact of an Increase of 3,000 U.S. Medical Graduates Per Year by 2015

*In the absence of an increase, the U.S. is likely to have about 972,000 active physicians in 2020.

*The increase in medical school graduates would add about 30,000 physicians by 2020, bringing the total supply to 1,002,000

*This is far less than the likely demand of between 1,027,000 and 1,240,000 physicians if services in 2020 are delivered as they were in 2002.

Source: AAMC Physician Workforce Research Conference, May 5-6, 2005

Experts at the AAMC meeting acknowledged that increasing the number of U.S. medical graduates will have no effect unless the number of residency training slots also is increased.   All increasing the number of U.S. medical graduates will do is reduce the number of residency slots taken by internationally trained physicians. The federal government will have to lift the cap it has set on the number of residency slots it will fund before the net number of physicians entering the workforce will increase.

But at least the physician supply experts now generally agree that there is a physician shortage. As they say in the self-help movement, you have to admit you have a problem before you can address it.

2. Managed Care Fizzled

We noted above that one of the main objectives of managed care was to reduce patient access to, and the use of, medical specialists.   The idea was that primary care physicians such as family doctors or internal medicine practitioners would take care of most things, and patients would only see specialists when absolutely necessary. Primary Care doctors would even be paid *not to* provide care or *not to* refer patients to specialists.   By giving them a fixed "per patient/per month" allowance, the less care doctors provided the more money they would make.

Unfortunately – or fortunately – this idea was completely out of tune with the American health care consumer and with the general arc of American society.   As Woody Allen said in another context, "The heart wants what it wants." People today want specialists – literally for the heart, in some instances.   Specialists are the ones who provide the really cool stuff that we need, or think we do – hip replacements, full body imaging scans, the latest drug therapies, botox and breast enhancements.

As long as we have the money to pay for these things, we are going to want them and we are going to get them.   And despite economic downturns such as the one we recently experienced, America remains a very rich country.   We want more stuff and we want better stuff.   In medicine, that means specialty care.   So the attempt to herd patients away from specialists and to limit access to medical services never caught fire as some experts thought that it would.   Go to your PPO doctor directory and you will see many doctors listed that you may choose from. You can still see those who aren't listed if you are willing to pay more. And in most cases, you won't need a referral from a primary care physician to get in.

3. We've been Training the Wrong Kinds of Physicians

The same experts alluded to above who believed that the U.S. had too many doctors also thought we had the wrong kind of doctors. About 68% of physicians in the U.S. today are specialists focusing on one or two body organs or systems. The rest are "generalists" focusing on the "whole person." As the old joke goes, a generalist is a doctor who treats what you have, while a specialist is a doctor who thinks you have what he treats. The two camps break out like this:

Generalists	Specialists
Family Practitioners	Anesthesiologists
General Internists	Cardiologists
Pediatricians	Cardiovascular surgeons
Total: 206,000	Dermatologists
(in active patient care only)	Gastroenterologists
	General Surgeons
	Neurologists
	Neuro Surgeons
	OB/GYNs
	Oncologists
	Ophthalmologists
	Orthopedic surgeons
	Otolaryngologists
	Pediatric subspecialists
	Psychiatrists
	Pulmonologists
	Radiologists
	Urologists
	Vascular surgeons
	And all others
	Total: 405,000
	(in active patient care only)

This imbalance between generalist and specialist physicians needed to be corrected, the experts thought, because the whole country was going to shift to a gatekeeper system, in which all patients would see a generalist doctor before they saw a specialist. The ideal ratio of generalists to specialists was thought to be 50/50. Half our doctors ought to be generalists, half specialists.

This message was widely broadcast to both medical educators and medical students during the early to mid-1990s. The Accreditation Council for Graduate Medical Education at this time suggested that specialist training be reduced by about 50%. Medical educators were convinced that for the sake of more appropriate, more efficient health care, they needed to educate and train more generalists.   Medical students were convinced that jobs for medical specialists were drying up and that they needed to go into general medicine.

For a few years in the early 1990s, this actually was the case.   Hospitals and medical groups everywhere went into a virtual frenzy trying to find primary care physicians, who they thought would be the key to the new system of health care. Control the primary care physician, they thought, and you would control the flow of patients.

When medical students completed their four years of medical school and had to choose a specialty in which to train, a much higher number began to choose one of the three generalist areas.   Fewer were available to go into specialty areas such as cardiology, as the following graph illustrates:

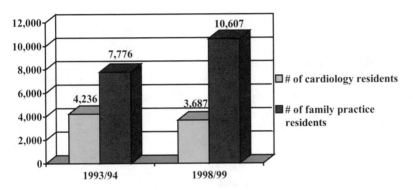

Source: Journal of the American Medical Association
(JAMA), Oct. 10, 1999

Medical educators were particularly vocal about steering medical students away from anesthesiology, since it was thought that managed care would greatly limit the number of surgeries performed in the U.S., thereby reducing the need for anesthesiologists.   According to the American Society of Anesthesiology, the number of residents completing training in anesthesiology dropped 44% between 1994 and 2000.

Unfortunately, at the precise moment that medical educators were funneling students into primary care, the need for specialists began to accelerate as the gatekeeper system largely failed to take hold and as the population began to age.

Our firm, which conducts over 2,600 physician search assignments each year, began to see a dramatic change in our business as the demand for physicians shifted from primary care doctors to specialists.   The following graph illustrates this trend:

Merritt, Hawkins & Associates Physician Search Assignments

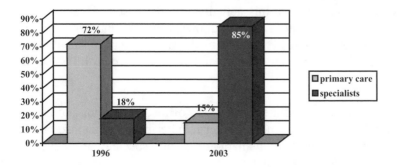

Source: Merritt, Hawkins & Associates

Today, the need for physicians is overwhelmingly in the specialty areas, with some exceptions (notably, rural districts – see Chapter 10.) Nevertheless, many medical educators are still committed to the proposition that 50% of all physicians trained should be generalists. The Department of Health and Human Services, for example, still sponsors a National Primary Care Week to bring more students into general medicine.

While generalists play a vital role, some of that role is being assumed by allied health professionals such as physician assistants and registered nurse practitioners (see Chapter 11.) There is no doubt we need primary care physicians, but the "50/50" rule is a fallacy. Medical students appear to have realized this and for a number of reasons – lifestyle and income among them – more medical graduates now are gravitating toward specialties and away from some areas of primary care (family practice, in particular.)

4. We're Getting Older – and Fatter – and There's More of Us

Here's the biggie. Like many industrialized countries, the United States has an aging population. The number of people 65 years old and older will double in the next 30 years, from 35 million to 70 million, according to the U.S. Census Bureau. The number of people 85 and older also will double, from 5 million to 10 million. Florida is now the oldest state in the union, followed by West Virginia, Pennsylvania, Rhode Island and Maine (the youngest states are Alaska, Utah, Texas, Georgia and Colorado.) Although some states will remain younger than others, the Census Bureau projects that by 2030 the population of the entire country will be as old as the population of Florida is now.

Older people use medical services at a higher rate than younger people. A much higher rate. In fact, people 66 years and older see a physician about three times more often each year than people 35 or younger (see below.)

Annual doctor visits by age

Age	Doctors visits per year
66 & older	6.0
46-65	5.4
36-45	3.5
25-35	2.2
16-24	1.5
0-15	2.0
Per population average	3.0

Source: National Ambulatory Healthcare Administration

According to the Centers for Disease Control and Prevention (CDC), the rate of doctor visits by Americans age 45 and older increased 17% from 1992 to 2001. About 53% of patients visiting the doctor in 2001 were over the age of 45, up from 26% in 1992, the CDC reports. Seniors and older Baby Boomers are visiting the doctor more often to manage multiple chronic conditions, obtain newly available drugs and seek preventive care.

Older people not only visit the doctor more often than younger people, they also require a higher rate of surgery. According to the National Center for Health Statistics, the rate of inpatient surgery for elderly people is three times higher than for the general population:

**Rate of inpatient surgery,
Elderly population....4,469 per 100,000 pop.**

**Rate of inpatient surgery,
General population.....1,519 per 100,000 pop.**

Source: National Center for Health Statistics

The National Hospital Discharge Survey reported in 1999 that patients aged 65 and older comprised 12% of the population but constituted 40% of hospital discharges and 48% of inpatient days.

To some extent, the American health care system is a victim of its own success. Due to advances in surgery and treatment, patients with diseases such as leukemia and colon cancer survive longer, but they require more care. The National Cancer

Institute, as referenced in the March 24, 2004 edition of *The Wall Street Journal,* estimates there are over 9.6 million cancer survivors in the United States – many of them needing regular therapy.

In addition, older people are less willing to accept a diminished quality of life today. The "active elderly" create a huge demand for things like hip replacements and treatment for neurological disorders such as Alzheimer's. More doctors will be needed to meet this demand, particularly specialists.

We can't control the fact that we are all aging (not yet, anyway) but we can control how we eat and how we behave. Unfortunately, many Americans don't. Obesity increased 60% from 1991 to 2000 and nearly one-fourth of the U.S. population is obese, according to an article in the March 8, 2004 edition of *Modern Healthcare.* A recent CDC study found that $75 billion was expended on obesity related illnesses in 2003, and that $39 billion of this tab was picked up by government-funded Medicare and Medicaid. A CDC study referenced in the March 9, 2004 edition of *The Washington Post* projected that obesity would become the number one cause of death in the U.S. by 2004, with the toll surpassing 500,000 per year.

One physician we spoke to recently described doctors as "the repairers of America's social indiscretions," because much of what they do is address the damage caused by excess eating and drinking, or by anti-social behaviors such as violence, divorce and other promoters of poor health. Unfortunately, it is becoming increasingly clear that we are going to need more "repairers."

Not only is there more *to us,* there are more *of us.* The Census Bureau estimates the U.S. population will grow from 285 million people in 2000 to 335 million people by 2020. That is nearly equivalent to adding the population of England over a period of 20 years.

What could make things really scary is the advent of new health care problems for which we are not fully prepared. Should some new strain of infectious disease arise (something on the scale of AIDS or even more catastrophic), or should terrorists succeed in launching biologic disasters, we will be happy for every physician we have – and we'll will wish we had many more.

5. *Young Doctor Kildaire Is Not So Young*

We will take a closer look at older doctors in Chapter 4. Suffice it to say the physician population in the U.S. reflects the general population. It is getting older, and the days of negative population growth among doctors are not too far away.

6. *No More Slave Labor*

There is an old Bill Cosby routine in which the "Cos" – laid out in a hospital – wants to call out for a young physician-in-training, but is not sure what term to use. So he bellows, "Hey, you! Almost a doctor!"

The real term for "almost a doctor," of course, is "resident." Toward the end of medical school, medical students must decide what area they are going to specialize in. Some medical students select family practice, some internal medicine, others radiology or any one of the dozens of other medical specialties that exist today. They then are "matched" with some of the 700 plus hospitals around the country that have resident training programs. Most of these "teaching hospitals" are larger facilities located in urban centers. Most residency programs last for three or four years, after which some physicians pursue a fellowship for even more training.

As mentioned above, these hospitals obtain funds through the Medicare program to help pay for resident training – so the doctor you see today probably had at least part of his or her training paid for by your tax dollars. Residents are paid while they train – but not much. The average annual salary is between $30,000 - $40,000.

While they train, residents provide care to patients at typically swamped urban hospitals. Often, they see the poorest paying patients – Medicaid patients, the uninsured and illegal immigrants. They also work like dogs – 100-hour weeks have been the norm in recent years. That's a pretty good deal for the teaching hospitals – a steady, cheap labor force that takes care of a lot of the "less desirable" patients whom hospitals otherwise could not afford to see.

This labor force is by no means insignificant. There are some 100,000 medical residents in the U.S. manning the front lines of care in the nation's largest hospitals.

Now, would you like to have a young physician in training who already has worked 75 hours that week treating you or your parent or child? Or would you like to be that resident, knowing that you are exhausted and not really in condition to make critical judgments about your patients' care? Probably not.

That's why in 2002 a rule was put into effect that limits residents' working hours to 80 per week – and proposals are being floated to reduce resident hours even more. Eighty hours a week is still a high load, but much less than the 100 hours they were accustomed to. This was a wise move likely to reduce medical errors made by residents, and certain to improve the working conditions residents must endure. However, it also reduces the physician man hours residents provide by about 20%. It's tantamount to taking about 15,000 to 20,000 physicians away from America's busiest hospitals.

No one is sure at the moment who is going to fill this gap.

7. It's A Woman's World

There was a time when physicians were men and nurses were women. If current trends continue, the inverse may be true. While the trickle of men going into nursing is becoming a stream, the trickle of women going into medicine has become a flood.

We'll address this critical trend in more detail in Chapter 3. For now, consider that female physicians work about 18% fewer hours per week than male physicians.

8. Dr. Patel to the Rescue?

In the last 20 years, the number of physicians practicing in the United States has grown for one reason – physicians educated overseas have come here to practice in increasing numbers. The number of students coming out of *U.S. medical schools* has not changed in the last two decades, but the number of students from *international medical schools* who come here has. Today, close to 25% of all physicians involved in active patient care in the U.S. are international medical graduates (IMGs.)

Each year, about 18,500 students graduate from U.S. medical schools and choose residency training programs at hospitals around the country. These programs take about three to four years to complete. At the end of every year – right around summer when schools and colleges get out – a new "class" of residents emerges from these training programs and officially enters the work force. The 2003 residency class numbered about 23,000. That includes the roughly 18,500 graduates of U.S. medical schools who completed their residency training plus about 4,000 graduates of international medical schools – many of them from Asia.

These physicians are eligible to practice in the U.S. provided they have completed medical school overseas, have taken a series of tests to prove their international training was on a par with U.S. training, and have completed the medical exam all physicians must take in order to get a medical license (the three-part U.S. Medical License Exam, or USMLE). They also must complete a three to four year residency training program at a U.S. teaching hospital. Like U.S.-trained physicians, they provide care to patients while they train as residents, for a very modest wage. Often, they represent the best and brightest doctors their countries have to offer.

Some of these IMGs return to their home countries once they have finished their U.S. residency training programs. Others stay, and many of these take jobs in areas that the federal government has designated as "medically underserved." There are over 2,500 federally designated Health Professional Shortage Areas (HPSAs) in the U.S., with a combined population of over 35 million people.

Sometimes IMGs are only a stop-gap solution in these areas. Once they have practiced for several years in a medically underserved area, they obtain a green card, at which point they can work anywhere in the U.S. Some leave the underserved area and relocate to areas not considered underserved. Others stay and become the lynchpins of medical care in their communities.

Without internationally trained medical graduates, the physician shortage would be considerably worse than it is now. Many rural areas in particular would be in a state of crisis or near crisis.

It is apparent, however, that IMGs are not a long-term solution to the physician supply problem. Increasingly, they are not even a short-term solution because the supply of IMGs has dropped significantly in the last several years. There are two reasons for this. One is the imposition in the year 2000 of the Clinical Skills Assessment test (CSA). This is a test all physicians trained in non-U.S. or non-Canadian medical schools must take to obtain a license to practice medicine here. The test is intended to gauge the ability of IMGs to diagnosis patients – to understand what patients are telling them and to explain their diagnosis to the patient so that the patient understands. Starting in 2005, all medical students, U.S. trained, Canadian trained, and internationally trained, will have to take the CSA.

The test is accomplished with the use of actors who pretend to have certain maladies, which they describe to the physician being tested. The use of actors, and the test itself, are considered controversial.

Aside from the debate over whether it is valid to use actors to fake illnesses is a debate over the cost and location of the test. The test costs over $1,200, which can be a prohibitive amount for some IMGs. For several years, it was only given in Philadelphia, which created a very big logistical problem for many IMGs who had to travel from their home countries to take the test or from around the U.S.

Since the test was imposed, the number of IMGs applying to be "matched" to U.S. residencies programs has dropped 20%.

The other limiting factor is the after-effects of 9/11. Since the terrorist strike, fewer government agencies have been willing to sponsor IMGs for the special "waivers" they need. Without these waivers, most IMGs are obligated to return to their home countries. With a waiver, they can stay in the U.S. and practice medicine, provided they practice in a federally designated medically underserved area.

In order to get a waiver, IMGs must obtain a sponsorship through a government agency. In the past, the principal sponsoring agency has been the Department of Agriculture (USDA). The USDA no longer sponsors IMGs for waivers, citing security concerns, so waivers have become increasingly hard to come by. The Department of Health and Human Services (HHS) instituted a waiver program, but the parameters are so tight that few hospitals or medical clinics in underserved areas can benefit from it.

Between the Clinical Skills Assessment Test and 9/11, the pipeline of IMGs coming to America has been significantly constricted. We cannot count on internationally trained physicians to bail us out, nor should we. While IMGs are making key contributions to health care nationwide, the United States should produce a sufficient number of physicians to care for its own population.

9. Doctors Are Filling Out Forms

Next time you are at the doctor's office, fuming because your appointment is running late, don't blame the physician for lingering on the golf course. As likely as not, he or she is being delayed by bureaucracy of one kind or another, not by a tough approach shot.

Physicians have to complete an increasing amount of paperwork today to ensure they are complying with government regulations, to cover their behinds so they don't get sued for malpractice, and to ensure that they get paid by insurance companies and the government. A recent American Hospital Association study indicates that physicians now spend one hour on paperwork for each hour they spend seeing patients.

Consider that the U.S. tax code runs to 11,000 pages. The Medicare rule book which doctors have to follow, by contrast, runs to 130,000 pages. For doctors, every day is like April 14, in terms of unwanted paperwork.

If physicians spend half their time filling out forms then you have to train twice as many physicians as you really need to get the job done. It's hoped that modern information technology will alleviate this problem, but so far the layers of bureaucracy being added to medicine are outstripping the ability of technology to deal with them.

10. Physicians Don't Practice Like They Used To

Numbers don't tell the whole story when it comes to physician supply. It is not just *how many* physicians there are that determines the adequacy or inadequacy of physician supply. What also is important is *how physicians practice medicine*. Physicians being trained today don't practice the same way as "old school" physicians do. This is largely the subject of Chapter 4. For the time being, let's just say that one younger physician entering the work force does not necessarily replace one older physician leaving the work force.

11. Technology Drives Demand

A generation or so ago, when you told the doctor you had a headache, there wasn't a whole lot he could do about it. "Take two aspirin and call me in the morning" became a cliché for a reason. The treatment options open to physicians just ten years ago were limited relative to what is available today. This is particularly true in three areas: diagnostics, surgery, and therapeutic drugs.

Today, diagnostic imaging – what used to be called radiology – is at the forefront of medicine. When it comes to detecting cancer or performing surgery or just about any other medical procedure, nothing can happen without a picture or image telling physicians what the problem is and where it is. The machines that capture these images – Computed Tomography (CT) scanners, Magnetic Resonance Imagers (MRI), Positron Emission Tomography (PET) scanners, mammography scanners, ultrasound – continue to proliferate. The old standby in imaging – the x-ray – also remains highly utilized. In fact, Medicare spending on diagnostic imaging has increased 100% since 1993, according to an article in the April 12, 2004 edition of *American Medical News.*

Hospital use of MRI and CT has grown 7.5% per year since 1996, according to an article in the December 15, 2002 edition of the *Minneapolis Star Tribune,* and the consulting firm Solucient reports that demand for imaging services will increase 67% between 2002 and 2007.

Greater sophistication in diagnosis is complemented by greater surgical sophistication. Knee and hip replacements, cardiac catheterization, non-invasive surgical techniques, transplantation – the options when it comes to operating are becoming limitless.

Perhaps the most visible leap in medical technology and in the variety of its application has been in pharmacology. Advertising for specific drugs used to be a rarity on television. Now, direct to consumer drug ads are ubiquitous on TV, magazines and other media. Viagra is the most visible of these new drug therapies, but there are many others that address both physical and psychological disorders. The new Medicare bill expanding drug benefits for seniors will only accelerate the use of prescription drugs.

Consider that the number of prescriptions written in the U.S. has almost doubled in the last four years alone.

Number of Annual Drug Prescriptions/U.S.

1998......1.2 billion
2002......2.1 billion
Total U.S. prescription drug sales
2003......$216.4 billion

Source: IMS Health/Modern Physician, 2/18/04

When a new diagnostic technique, a less invasive surgical procedure, or a "wonder drug" is introduced, patients almost invariably embrace them. "Virtual colonoscopy" offers a good example. Using non-invasive imaging, radiologists can check patients for colon cancer in a manner much more comfortable than the traditional style of colonoscopy, in which a tube must be inserted into the patient's rectum. Patients who were reluctant to submit to the old style of diagnostic technique are very likely to embrace the new style in increasing numbers. So technology creates more demand for medical services than previously existed.

It requires physicians, of course, (specialists, in particular) to carry out these diagnostic and surgical techniques and to prescribe the new generation of drugs. The more that can be done in medicine, the more physicians are needed to do it. It only takes one doctor to say, "Take two aspirin and call me in the morning." But when a patient has a headache today, it may take a family physician to send him to a neurologist, who then may send him to a radiologist for a CT scan, who then may have to bring in a neurosurgeon or an oncologist if cancer is involved, who then will bring in an anesthesiologist should surgery be necessary. In addition to involving five or six different types of doctors, the process may involve a large team of nurses, technologists, lab specialists and therapists.

No wonder health care now employs more people than any other part of the private sector – over 10 million people. And it still does not employ enough people to get the job done.

Not nearly enough.

12. *An Old Standby – Maldistribution*

We have discussed why *how physicians practice* is almost as important as how many physicians there are. Of course, *where physicians practice* also is a critical factor in the physician supply equation.

The places where physicians train (medical schools and teaching hospitals) are mostly located in big cities. When physicians complete their training they often look to settle in the area where they trained, or in some other urban center that offers the lifestyle amenities most highly educated professionals seek – restaurants, art galleries, movie theaters, book stores, opera companies, etc.

There are not many opera companies in Small Town America, and there are not many physicians, either. Over 20% of the population is classified as rural by the U.S. Census Bureau, but less than 11% of practicing physicians are located in rural areas. The concentration of physicians in urban areas has existed for several generations and is driven in part by the move toward specialization in medicine. Specialists generally need to be near larger population centers. It takes some 25,000 people to support one oncologist, but only about 4,000 people to support one family physician.

Following is a graph showing states with the most physicians per capita, and states with the fewest physicians per capita:

Non Federal Physicians per 100,000 Population

States with the most physicians per capita		*States with the fewest physicians per capita*	
1.	District of Columbia – 718	51.	Idaho – 178
2.	Massachusetts – 448	50.	Mississippi – 181
3.	New York – 409	49.	Oklahoma – 184
4.	Maryland – 406	48.	Alaska – 194
5.	Connecticut – 385	47.	Nevada – 196
6.	Vermont – 375	46.	Wyoming – 197
7.	Rhode Island – 357	45.	Iowa – 199
8.	New Jersey – 323	44.	Arkansas – 208
9.	Pennsylvania – 318	43.	South Dakota – 214
10.	Hawaii – 300	42.	Texas – 217

Source: AMA Physician Masterfile as referenced in the December 23, 2002 edition of Modern Healthcare

The rural population is aging more rapidly than the general population and it is specialists who provide the treatments and procedures that many older people need. Access to specialists – and, in many cases, to generalists, as well – is limited in rural areas, and even if the overall supply of physicians increases, this will continue to be the case. For the same reasons you don't find many architects, scientists, engineers, lawyers, or computer programmers in small towns, you don't find very many physicians. Most of these people simply prefer to live in large or mid-sized communities.

Rising malpractice rates also contribute to the maldistribution of physicians. Physicians tend to leave high malpractice areas to find more sheltered areas. West Virginia, for example, recently experienced an exodus of doctors from the state as malpractice rates rose, with over 100 physicians leaving in less than one year. Doctors are now starting to move back to West Virginia since it instituted tort reform.

There is an additional and perhaps insurmountable reason why rural areas are likely to be physician poor for a long time – but you'll need to read Chapter 10 to find out what it is.

The Doctor Is Out

The combined effect of these twelve trends will be marginal access to physicians and greater costs to health care consumers (you and me.) Unlike most professionals, physicians don't set their own fees. These are determined by "third party payors" such as insurance companies and the federal government, through Medicare and Medicaid. When it comes to what they can charge, physicians have to either take what payors give them, or leave it.

Or do they? You may have heard or read about a trend called "boutique medicine." This is a style of medicine in which patients pay doctors a lump annual sum to provide them with medical care. It's direct physician-to-patient contracting. No insurer or third party payor is involved. You also may have visited physicians who no longer accept insurance of any kind – it is cash only, or find another doctor. This is the old style of "fee-for-service" medicine that was in vogue before the days of managed care and discounted payment plans such as PPOs.

Back in Chapter 1 we observed that many physicians surveyed are not seeing Medicaid patients. Others won't see Medicare patients. When there are plenty of patients and few doctors, doctors can afford to pick and choose the patients they see. They also don't have to accept lower reimbursement rates from insurance companies. That means insurance companies will have to pay more to keep doctors participating in their plans. The insurance companies then will charge their customers more. For the most part, their customers are employers, who are finding it hard to pay for rising health insurance costs. Increasingly, employers are obliged to pass some of these costs on to their employees, in the form of higher deductibles and higher co-pays.

It's a simple matter of supply and demand. A small supply of physicians + a greater demand for their services = higher costs.

Some people think that the laws of supply and demand don't apply to health care. They do. Keep a close track of what you are spending on physician services in the next few years if you don't agree.

The X Factor

Is there anything that can change this scenario, anything that will lead to a more appropriate balance between the supply and demand for physicians in the next 10 to 15 years?

The short answer is no. There is no pressing political will at present to build more medical schools or create new residency training programs – a subject we discuss in more detail in Chapter 12 – and even if there were, the supply of physicians can't be significantly altered overnight.

The only event that could alter the picture would be a sudden decrease in demand for the medical services physicians provide. As referenced above, demand for medical care is going nowhere but up – unless, and only unless, the economy goes down. In the face of a protracted recession or an outright depression (the X factor), the wealth that promotes health that in turn drives the need for doctors will disappear. Much of the new diagnostic testing, the new surgical procedures, and the new drugs alluded to earlier will be beyond the price range of the majority and the need for physicians – specialists, in particular – will decline.

However, at no time since the Great Depression has the economy significantly dampened demand for health care services. Health care commonly is thought of as recession proof, because people need it whether the economy is booming or slumping.

The most recent recession saw net job losses in many industries. Hospitals, medical groups and other health care providers, by contrast, couldn't hire people fast enough. As Merritt, Hawkins & Associates' 2005 Survey of Hospital Physician Recruiting Trends illustrates, the rush to recruit physicians continues today. The survey shows that, as of the spring of 2005, 88% of hospitals of all sizes were recruiting physicians. Larger hospitals, however, are virtually in continuous physician recruiting mode. The survey indicates that 95% of hospitals of 101 – 200 beds are recruiting physicians and that 98% of hospitals of 201 beds or more are recruiting physicians (a copy of this survey can be found at the end of this book.)

Should the U.S. economy exhibit its customary strength in the next 15 years, demand for health services will continue to rise, which means we will need more physicians. More physicians are just what we will not have, however. In fact, we will have fewer.

Why? Well, for one thing, young doctors are in love -- which is the subject of Chapter 3.

Chapter 3:
Young Doctors in Love

"A youth is to be regarded with respect. How do we know that his future will not be equal to our present?" -- Confucius

It's true, young doctors are in love. They are in love with their spouses, their kids, and what is commonly referred to as their "quality of life."

Does this make them any different from doctors who trained 15, 20, or 25 years ago? Yes, it does, in a way that is dramatically affecting the supply of physicians. Generation X and Y doctors – those who were born any time after 1964 or so – have a different perspective on medicine than do the "Old School" physicians who preceded them in the profession.

Younger physicians, to borrow Martha Stewart's phrase, want to "have it all." Family, career, travel, hobbies. Just like other highly trained professionals, they want to enjoy a good living but still get to see their kids' baseball games and piano recitals, still go on regular vacations, still dabble in hobbies, still have a world separate from medicine they can call their own.

This represents a significant break from the traditional culture of American medical practice. For "Old School" physicians there often is little distinction between one's personal and professional life. You are a physician 24/7. The practice comes first, even if it means 80 to 100 hour weeks and even if family life has to be sacrificed. But don't take our word for it – ask any Old School physician's wife – his *first* wife, that is (and we say *his* for a reason, which we will get to presently.)

This new attitude among young doctors is a positive development in many ways. Physicians deserve to have a private life like anyone else, and it can be argued that well adjusted, well-balanced physicians are likely to provide a higher level of care than physicians who do not enjoy a work/life balance.

It does, however, inhibit the total number of physician man hours and it reduces the number of patients seen.

Working for the Man

It is not too difficult to explain why younger physicians often have a different attitude toward medicine than older ones – and it's not because the younger generation is lazy or less committed than their elders.

The main reason is that medicine has changed in the last 15 to 20 years. When Old School physicians joined the profession they enjoyed an exalted status reflected in television shows such as "Ben Casey," "Dr. Kildaire," and "Marcus Welby, M.D." Patients didn't question the doctor's orders and insurance companies did not question how doctors practiced. A physician would perform a service and the insurance company would pay him for that service. It was the Golden Age of Fee-For-Service Medicine.

Just as important, physicians in the Golden Age were their own bosses. Typically, they would come out of training, select a practice location, and "hang up a shingle." Or they might join a relative or family friend in practice. They were essentially small business operators – the more they worked, the more patients they saw, the more money they earned.

Perhaps best of all, they knew their patients. An Old School doctor, particularly one in family practice, might treat a patient most of his or her life, and treat the patient's children and maybe even his or her grandchildren. There was such a thing as physician/patient loyalty. And for the most part, physicians didn't have to worry about their patients becoming their adversaries in court.

None of this is true of physicians today. The usual career path for physicians today entails the following:

- 12 years of primary and secondary education…3.5 grade average or higher, 1400 SATs or higher

- 4 years of college/university…pre-med courses: math, chemistry, biology, 3.5 grade average or higher

- 4 years of medical school…rigorous scientific training

- 3-4 years of residency training…hands on doctoring at a teaching hospital. No sleep. Low pay. Lives are in your hands. Are we having fun yet?

- 1-2 years of fellowship training. Learn how to operate on a child's brain or transplant a heart. Don't try this at home.

Congratulations, you're a doctor. You're ready for your first job. You also are likely to be $100,000 in debt. Medical education and training are expensive

Level of Educational Debt
Among Graduating Medical Students

Class of 2003

Average debt	$109,457
$100,000 or more	58%
$150,000 or more	25.4%
$200,000 or more	7.5%

Source: Assn. of American Medical Colleges 2003 Graduating Questionnaire

Today, the great majority of physicians enter the workforce as employees – not independent business people running their own show. For the most part, they work for other physicians in a group practice. They collect a paycheck or they are guaranteed to make a certain amount by a medical group or a hospital. They also may earn a bonus for reaching certain goals, such as a percentage of the fees collected from the patients they see.

But seeing patients – or a greater number of them – may not impact their earnings much. Why? Because certain patients are covered by insurance plans that don't pay very well. Sometimes the claims doctors submit to insurance plans are rejected because the plans may not cover the service or procedure the doctor provided. Sometimes the claims are rejected because someone at the insurance company (though usually not a physician) determined that what the doctor did was either unnecessary or not appropriate. The doctor didn't follow the "treatment protocol" dictated by the plan. That's what is known as "cookbook medicine." Follow the recipe, doctor, or don't get paid. Sometimes, it's not the number of patients you see, but their ability to pay, that results in a higher income.

The patients the physician sees will come to her not because she's particularly well trained, or because they have heard of her, or knew her daddy, but because she is "part of their insurance plan." The physician's group has negotiated with a Preferred Provider Organization (PPO) and it has accepted the discounted reimbursement rates they offer in exchange for the patients they are likely to see who are signed up with the PPO. When the patient's company changes PPOs, the patient will drop the physician if her group does not participate in the new PPO. Should the group decide to drop the PPO the patient is on, the patient will find another physician who still participates in the plan.

Continuity – an important element in quality of care – often is lost in contemporary medicine. Physician/patient loyalty often is lacking.

Patients and physicians still can get to know one another very well. Unfortunately, it generally happens in court. Patients are increasingly likely to sue their doctors, and the settlements they receive are getting larger.

By the time young physicians complete their residency training, they generally know the score. They have dealt with the hassles of managed medicine and they may even have been the target of a malpractice suit themselves. They also have dealt with patients who are outright disrespectful and – thanks to all the medical information and misinformation to be found on the Internet – think they know more about a particular ailment or condition than the doctor does. Occasionally – very occasionally – they are right.

The result is an alarmingly high level of disillusionment. Merritt, Hawkins & Associates conducts a survey every other year of residents completing their final year of training. Following is one of the questions we asked:

If you had your career to plan again, would you study medicine or would you select another field?

	2001	2003
Study medicine	95%	74%
Select another field	5%	26%

Source: Merritt, Hawkins & Associates 2004 Survey of Final Year Medical Residents

Rather than being happy and enthusiastic about entering their chosen profession, as they should be, one in four young physicians would like to be doing something else. The word about the "hassle factors" of medicine – the long, expensive training cycle, managed care, malpractice, etc. – has filtered out to the public at large.   For six years in a row (1996-2002) applications to medical school declined as fewer of our best and brightest college graduates were attracted to the medical profession. Applications went up again in 2003 but are still well below previous highs.

Applicants to Medical School

1996	2002
47,000	33,501

Source: Association of American Medical Colleges

What was considered a "way of life" for Old School Physicians who enjoyed professional autonomy, patient loyalty and respect, and a direct correlation between how hard they worked and how much they were paid, now is considered a job by many younger physicians. Medicine as a job means set hours, regular pay, vacations and a greater degree of emotional and physical detachment than does medicine as a way of life.

One symptom of this is that young physicians are becoming increasingly nomadic. According to an article published in the May 22, 2001 issue of *The New York Times,* before 1990 only one to two percent of physicians changed jobs throughout a 20 year career. Now, more than 10 percent of physicians change jobs in any given year. The average physician who entered practice after 1990 was likely to have had at least three jobs by 2000.

It is not that younger physicians are any less capable than their predecessors. On the contrary, physicians today are very well trained and can do more for their patients than any other generation of physicians could.

Nevertheless, one physician entering practice today does not equal one Old School physicians leaving medicine from a pure man power point of view. Indeed, we have found that it sometimes takes two younger doctors to replace one older one.

You Go, Girl

There is another difference between Generation X and Y physicians and the Old School – a big difference. Increasingly, the doctor of today is a woman. The Association of American Medical Colleges announced in 2003 that for the first time ever the number of women applying to medical school was greater than the number of men. The number of women *accepted* into medical school reached 49% in 2003.

Female physicians already dominate the ranks of some residency programs and they make up a significant percentage of others (see below)

Percent of Residents Who Are Female

OB/GYN	68%
Pediatrics	65%
Dermatology	54%
Psychiatry	49%
Family Practice	47%
Pathology	47%
Internal Medicine	40%
Radiology	25%
General Surgery	21%

Source: Association of American Medical Colleges

Not only is the physician of the future likely to be a woman, she is likely to be an Asian-American woman. The number of Asian-American women enrolled in medical school has increased by more than 50% to 5,994 students in 2001, up from 3,928 in 1992, according to the Association of American Medical Colleges.

Why are more women seeking careers in medicine? Because they can. Attitudes have changed and women interested in health care no longer are confined to nursing. Some women actually are choosing medicine because they see it as a way to have a balanced lifestyle!

Consider the comments of a female medical student quoted in a December, 2003 issue of the *Los Angeles Times* ("More Women Seeking a Healthy Future in Medicine"):

"One of the things that's great about medicine is the flexibility. I'm considering going into emergency medicine, and that has a wonderful lifestyle if you're considering having a family."

Flexibility? Wonderful lifestyle? These are concepts foreign to Old School physicians but common among younger physicians today.

Again, this change is mostly for the good. Half of all people are women, so why shouldn't half of all physicians be women? In addition, there is some evidence that female physicians spend more time with patients than do male physicians and they are thought to display a more empathetic attitude. The perception definitely exists that women prefer to see female OB/GYNs – to the detriment of some male OBs who feel they are passed over for jobs.

That said, there is no question that the influx of women into medicine is having and will have an enormous inhibiting effect on overall physician supply. As referenced in Chapter 2, female physicians work 18% fewer hours per week than male physicians, largely due to their dual role as professionals and mothers.

An old science fiction movie went by the provocative title, *"Mars Needs Women."* Well, medicine needs women – even more of them.

And more men, too.

Chapter Four:
The Old School's Last Stand

"It takes five years to learn how to operate, and twenty years to learn when not to." -- An old medical school saying.

Suppose you needed a hip replaced or your heart repaired. Who would be the best qualified physician to perform surgical procedures so vital to your well being, and perhaps to your very existence?

The best answer is, a doctor who had done these types of procedures before. Many times before.

Evidence is mounting that the physicians who achieve the best surgical outcomes are the ones who have done a particular procedure the most. According to a study published in the November, 27, 2003 issue of the *New England Journal of Medicine,* a patient was 24% more likely to die from complications during lung resection or within 30 days after the operation if the surgeon performed fewer than seven of the procedures annually, as compared to a surgeon who does more than 17 a year. Other studies also point to physician experience as a key factor in achieving positive outcomes in surgery.

It's a pretty simple concept that we learn at the earliest age from parents or instructors trying to teach us a new skill: Practice makes perfect.

The best physician for the job, then, may not be the one just out of the internationally renowned fellowship program or a physician affiliated with a world famous hospital. It may simply be the older doc who's been around the block (or the knee, or the heart) a few times.

Logic suggests that the same principle holds true for diagnostic physicians such as radiologists or family practitioners. Having looked at hundreds of thousands of x-rays, an experienced radiologist may see a malignancy where a less experienced one sees healthy bone. And an experienced family practitioner may hear a potentially dangerous heart murmur where a less experienced one hears a regular heart beat.

Experience does not always equate to quality when it comes to physicians, but it appears to be the best predictor of good outcomes that we have.

The good news is that there are a lot of experienced physicians in the United States that patients can turn to. According to the American Medical Association, 38% of all physicians in the U.S. are 50 years old or older. Close to one-third (30%) are 55 and older.

The bad news is that a lot of these doctors are disillusioned with the way medicine is practiced today and are looking to get out. The defection of older physicians from medicine is going to be a major contributing factor to the doctor shortage in the next 15 years. Not only will we have fewer physicians, but the quality of those we do have will suffer when the experienced, knowledgeable vets bow out. As brilliant and well trained as many young physicians are, it is hard to beat experience in just about any endeavor.

To understand why the flight of older physicians from medicine matters, it's important to consider that old doctors, like old soldiers, don't die…they just fade away. At least, they used to.

One reason it is difficult to track the precise moment that older physicians retire is that often there is no such precise moment. A business executive retires after 30 years, gets his gold watch, and is no longer on the payroll. Professionals in most other fields generally make a clean break when it comes time to retire. One day they are accountants, they next day they are not.

Physicians, by contrast, usually do a slow fade out. They hold onto their medical licenses and see a diminishing amount of patients, often well into their seventies or even their eighties. They may only be working 20 hours a week, and only seeing established patients that they have seen for many years, but they are still practicing, still making a contribution to patient care.

That will not be the pattern in coming years, and is less frequently the pattern today. Why? For one thing, patient loyalty is not what it once was. As explained in the previous chapter, patients follow their insurance plans, they don't follow their physicians. So the old patient who has been with the old doctor forever is a vanishing paradigm. The emotional ties that bound physicians to medicine are weakening.

But of more importance is the fact that older physicians don't like the rules by which medicine is played today. They don't like the bureaucracy, they don't like the lack of autonomy, and they don't like having targets on their backs when it comes to plaintiffs and their attorneys seeking big paydays in court. The satisfaction they received from taking care of patients is no longer commensurate with the attending hassles of practicing medicine.

Consider the results of a survey of 436 physicians between the ages of 50 – 65 that Merritt, Hawkins & Associates conducted in November, 2003. We asked physicians in this age group a variety of questions, including the following:

In the last five years, have you found the practice of medicine to be more satisfying, less satisfying, or has your satisfaction level remained the same?

More satisfying	9%
Less satisfying	76%
The same	15%

What is your greatest source of professional frustration?

Long hours	10%
Malpractice worries	28%
Managed care	16%
Medicare/ Medicaid regulations	13%
Pressure of running a business	10%
Patient attitudes today	5%
Other	9%
N/A	9%

In the next one to three years, do you plan to:

Retire	8%
Seek a medical job in a non-clinical setting	10%
Seek a job or business in a non-medical field	3%
Work locum tenens	6%
Close practice to new patients significantly reduce workload	17%
Continue as you are	49%
Other	7%

The first point to keep in mind when evaluating this survey is that the group we targeted represents a very large number of physicians. Over 250,000 physicians are between the ages of 50 and 65, according to the AMA. Often, doctors in this age group are the "work horses" of the hospital medical staff – old school physicians who see a lot of patients and work a lot of hours. In addition, due to their training and experience, they provide some of the best patient care available anywhere in the world.

We cannot afford to lose these physicians, but that is just what is going to happen.

Add up the responses to the final question above and you'll see that 51% of physicians 50 to 65 years old plan to either stop seeing patients in the next one to three years, reduce the number of patients they see, or pursue some other option rather than practicing as they are.

Due in part to the stock market, which suffered after the dot-com bust, most of these physicians cannot afford to retire immediately. However, many of them still are looking for a way out of traditional medical practice. Ten percent indicate they will seek medical jobs in non-clinical settings. This means they will continue to work in health care, but will not be seeing patients. Many such jobs are available, in areas such hospital or medical group management, or in research, or with one of the many growing pharmaceutical companies that hire physicians as consultants or managers. Three percent will seek opportunities in a non-medical field. Including those planning to retire, 21% of physicians surveyed indicated they will stop seeing patients in the next one to three years.

An additional six percent indicated they will work on a "locum tenens" basis. This means they will work on temporary assignments, often part-time (see chapter 8 for a fuller explanation of temporary doctors.) Seventeen percent indicated they will either stop seeing new patients or significantly reduce the number of patients they see. Eleven percent of those surveyed already have closed their practices to new patients.

It is true that people don't always do what they say they are going to do in surveys. But let's presume for the sake of argument that just 10% of physicians between the ages of 50 and 65 stop seeing patients in the next one to three years, not the 21% who say they will in the survey. And let's discount for a moment the diminishing effect on overall physician supply of older physicians who plan to stop seeing new patients or significantly reduce the number of patients they see.

The effect on patient care of a defection of even 10% of these veteran physicians from medicine would be enormous. According to the Medical Group Management Association, the average annual number of patient office visits handled by physicians of all types is 2,100. Should 10% of all physicians age 50 – 65 -- some 25,000 doctors – stop seeing patients, 52,000,000 annual patient visits will have to be absorbed by remaining physicians.

It is important to stress again that many of these older physicians are in their peak years, in terms of the number of patients they see. They have built up practices over the course of two decades or more and are at full capacity. As referenced above, when one of these physicians leaves the field of medicine, it can take more than one younger physician to replace him.

This is one point on which older physicians themselves are clearly undivided. Consider the responses to the following question from Merritt, Hawkins & Associates' Survey of physicians 50 – 65 Years Old.

Consider the dedication and work ethic of physicians coming out of training today. Are physicians being trained today?

Less dedicated and hard working than physicians who entered medicine when you did?	64%
More dedicated and hard working than physicians who entered medicine when you did?	0%
Just as dedicated and hard working as physicians who entered medicine when you did?	29%
Other	5%
N/A	2%

It is telling to note that of the 436 physicians who answered the survey, not a single one indicated that physicians being trained today are more dedicated and hard working than those trained in the past. The following are remarks taken from a letter to the editor of the AMA publication *American Medical News*. The letter was submitted by a physician who had read a story in this publication regarding Merritt, Hawkins' survey of older doctors.

"I am 57 years old and have been practicing maternal fetal medicine as well as obstetrics and gynecology for more than 20 years. Indeed, I can readily attest to the fact that many of today's (Generation X) doctors are "9 to 5ers." They do not want to get out of bed at 2 a.m. to see their patients. Moreover, it is true for both male and female doctors. I put in about 60 to 70 hours a week. When my patients need me, I'm there. Not so with the "9 to 5ers."

Source: American Medical News, March 8, 2004.

Here is another letter to the editor that appeared in the same issue, written by a younger physician:

"To those doctors who came before me I say: You are right. I am less hard working and dedicated to medicine than you are. I am not available to my patients at all hours. I do not practice obstetrics. I do not accept frequent call and after hours responsibilities. Some superheroes do it all (God help the spouses and families of the superheroes.) We all have strengths and weaknesses; let's support each other and strive for our best as a team."

In previous generations, older, "workhorse" doctors could be counted on to practice medicine long after 55. That is not the case today and will not be the case in the future. Many older physicians will retire as soon as they can afford to, or will opt out of traditional patient care in some other way. As a result, we will soon reach a point where the number of physicians leaving medicine will exceed those entering the field, as the chart below indicates.

Projected Physician Attrition / Exits to Exceed Entrants

	2020
Physicians dying or retiring annually	23,000
U.S. trained physicians entering the workforce annually	16,000 – 18,500
IMGs entering the workforce	Unknown

Physician population will reach negative growth sometime in the next 10 to 15 years.

Source: MGT of America

Because demand for medical services is rising and the supply of physicians falling, it is important now and will be even more import in the future that medicine have its advocates – people who will encourage our most promising students to enter this vital field.   But who will those advocates be?

The Demise of the Medical Family

Just as there are many "military families" in the U.S. there also are many "medical families."   In military families, several generations have served in the U.S. Armed Forces, sometimes going back to the Civil War or farther.   Today's Lt. Colonel looks back on the career of an uncle who served in WWII and offers that as a key factor in his decision to become a military officer.

Similarly, in medical families, one or more family members have been doctors for two or three generations or more. Talk to ten medical students today and five of them will point to a father, mother, uncle or aunt who is a physician and who inspired them to go into medicine.   That is one reason why it was such a breakthrough when women and minorities were able to enter the field and serve as role models for others. The best advocates for medicine as a career have always been other physicians.

It therefore is disturbing and alarming when older physicians, rather than advocating for the medical profession, actively warn young people away from it.

Consider these questions from our survey of physicians 50 to 65.

If you were starting out today, would you choose medicine as your career?

Yes   48%
No   52%

Would you encourage your children or other young people to choose medicine as a career today?

Yes   36%
No   64%

Over half of older doctors now wish they had not gone into medicine, according to the survey. Over six in ten would not encourage their children or other young people to become doctors.

Researchers use various models and formulas to calculate the projected need for physicians in the United States. None of them incorporate the effect one disillusioned physician has when he plants a seed of negatively about his profession in the mind of a young person. Many such seeds have been planted in recent years - - a troubling sign of a poor harvest in years to come.

Chapter Five:
What Doctors Make

A plumber hands a doctor his bill for fixing a leaky faucet.

"Six-hundred dollars!" the doctor exclaims. "That's ridiculous. I don't make that much as a physician."

"Neither did I," says the plumber, "when I was a physician."

Having read this far, we know what you are thinking. What do doctors (both young and old) have to complain about? They all make a ton of money, don't they?

Not exactly.

There are many types of physicians, as we have noted above. Some of them make very good incomes. Some of them are not particularly well paid relative to the time and money they put into becoming physicians, and relative to the time and stress required to be a physician.

We mentioned already that medical students are, on average, over $100,000 in debt by the time they graduate. One in four is over $150,000 in debt. This debt often grows during the three, four, or even five years medical graduates then spend in residency training or as fellows.

Physicians generally are in their late twenties or early thirties before they emerge from training and begin earning a truly professional income. Some of this income is siphoned off to service their high debt load. They frequently don't have time to "ramp up" financially in order to start a family, because their training years also are their prime child producing years. They start on the "road of life" late, in debt, and often with a child or two to raise.

If they are family physicians, internists, or pediatricians (i.e., if they provide "primary care") they likely will earn solid middle to upper middle class incomes. Primary care physicians just getting started will typically be offered salaries in the $120,000 – $130,000 range. If the community has an urgent need for a doctor, they may make somewhat more. If the community is in a resort area or some other highly desirable location they will make less. Primary care physicians in a mature practice usually earn between $130,000 – $180,000 annually, though there are experienced primary care doctors making less than this, and a very small percentage who make more.

Not a bad income, but hardly Bill Gates money by any stretch of the imagination. Primary care physicians, of which there are over 200,000 in active patient care, still have to sweat their mortgages, worry about college tuition for their kids, and plan carefully for retirement. They are by no means rich – at least not relative to successful business people, bankers, lawyers, or stock brokers. Ironically, successful physician recruiters sometimes earn more money than the physicians they recruit.

Specialists, by contrast, usually earn considerably more than primary care doctors, and a few even become millionaires.

In the past, when most doctors were independent contractors, there was not a great deal of data concerning their incomes. Since doctors mostly paid themselves, few organizations kept track of doctor pay. Now, however, many doctors are employed, and hospitals, medical groups, HMOs and other employers have a stake in knowing what doctors earn, so that they will know what to pay them. Consequently, a number of medical group associations, recruiting, and financial benefits organizations generate data tracking physician compensation.

Following is a break down of average annual physician compensation in a variety of specialties as determined by several of these organizations. These numbers are compiled every year and published in *Modern Healthcare*, a leading health care industry publication. The following numbers appeared in *Modern Healthcare's* July 19, 2004 edition. In addition, note that at the end of this book is a copy of Merritt, Hawkins & Associates' *2005 Review of Physician Recruiting Incentives*. The Review indicates the type of financial and other incentives that are being offered to recruit physicians by hospitals and medical groups. Numbers from Merritt, Hawkins & Associates' 2005 Review will be included in *Modern Healthcare's* 2005 breakdown of physician income. All numbers below, including Merritt, Hawkins & Associates', are from *Modern Healthcare's* 2004 compilation of physician income.

Anesthesiology

Medical Group Management Association (MGMA)	$341,407
Hay Group	$320,300
American Medical Group Association (AMGA)	$301,503
Merritt, Hawkins& Associates	$300,000
Hospital & Healthcare Compensation Services (HHCS)	$291,627
Sullivan, Cotter & Associates	$258,277
Warren Surveys	N/A

Cardiology (non-invasive)

Hay Group	$366,700
Medical Group Management Association (MGMA)	$362,497

American Medical Group Association (AMGA)	$345,254
Hospital & Healthcare Compensation Services (HHCS)	$335,577
Merritt, Hawkins & Associates	$292,000
Sullivan, Cotter & Associates	$276,145
Warren Surveys	$270,764

Emergency Medicine

Merritt, Hawkins & Associates	$236,000
Medical Group Management Association (MGMA)	$226,561
American Medical Group Association (AMGA)	$219,860
Hay Group	$216,100
Sullivan, Cotter & Associates	$205,104
Hospital & Healthcare Compensation Services (HHCS)	$167,621
Warren Surveys	N/A

Family Practice

Medical Group Management Association (MGMA)	$166,301
American Medical Group Association (AMGA)	$166,162
Hospital & Healthcare Compensation Services (HHCS)	$158,143
Sullivan, Cotter & Associates	$155,658
Hay Group	$154,900
Warren Surveys	$151,051
Merritt, Hawkins & Associates	$146,000

General Surgery

American Medical Group Association (AMGA)	$297,208
Medical Group Management Association (MGMA)	$291,684
Sullivan, Cotter & Associates	$261,341
Merritt, Hawkins & Associates	$248,000
Hospital & Healthcare Compensation Services (HHCS)	$234,530

| Warren Surveys | $232,701 |
| Hay Group | $232,500 |

Internal Medicine

Hay Group	$177,800
Medical Group Management Association (MGMA)	$172,342
American Medical Group Association (AMGA)	$162,130
Hospital & Healthcare Compensation Services (HHCS)	$160,631
Sullivan, Cotter & Associates	$157,611
Warren Surveys	$157,112
Merritt, Hawkins & Associates	$152,000

Neurology

Hay Group	$239,000
Medical Group Management Association (MGMA)	$219,912
American Medical Group Association (AMGA)	$205,992
Merritt, Hawkins & Associates	$191,000
Hospital & Healthcare Compensation Services (HHCS)	$182,348
Warren Surveys	$178,403
Sullivan, Cotter & Associates	$169,304

OB/GYN

Hay Group	$252,300
Medical Group Management Association (MGMA)	$261,073
American Medical Group Association (AMGA)	$266,245
Merritt, Hawkins & Associates	$242,000
Hospital & Healthcare Compensation Services (HHCS)	$233,343
Warren Surveys	$237,066
Sullivan, Cotter & Associates	$222,625

Oncology

Medical Group Management Association (MGMA)	$346,614
Merritt, Hawkins & Associates	$276,000
American Medical Group Association (AMGA)	$273,160
Hospital & Healthcare Compensation Services (HHCS)	$249,512
Sullivan, Cotter & Associates	$233,293
Hay Group	$228,900
Warren Surveys	$228,141

Pathology

Medical Group Management Association (MGMA)	$324,827
Hay Group	$268,800
American Medical Group Association (AMGA)	$256,680
Hospital & Healthcare Compensation Services (HHCS)	$238,623
Sullivan, Cotter & Associates	$226,921
Warren Surveys	$213,693
Merritt, Hawkins & Associates	N/A

Pediatrics

Medical Group Management Association (MGMA)	$172,058
American Medical Group Association (AMGA)	$166,069
Hay Group	$162,400
Warren Surveys	$153,421
Sullivan, Cotter & Associates	$148,027
Merritt, Hawkins & Associates	$144,000
Hospital & Healthcare Compensation Services (HHCS)	$141,402

Psychiatry

Medical Group Management Association (MGMA)	$164,221
Merritt, Hawkins & Associates	$162,000
Hay Group	$160,400
American Medical Group Association (AMGA)	$159,703
Warren Surveys	$157,148
Sullivan, Cotter & Associates	$142,685
Hospital & Healthcare Compensation Services (HHCS)	$131,688

Radiology

Medical Group Management Association (MGMA)	$386,214
American Medical Group Association (AMGA)	$332,160
Hospital & Healthcare Compensation Services (HHCS)	$325,829
Merritt, Hawkins & Associates	$317,000
Hay Group	$285,500
Sullivan, Cotter & Associates	$274,357
Warren Surveys	$192,457

Urology

Medical Group Management Association (MGMA)	$334,019
American Medical Group Association (AMGA)	$321,669
Hospital & Healthcare Compensation Services (HHCS)	$299,719
Merritt, Hawkins & Associates	$277,000
Sullivan, Cotter & Associates	$253,903
Hay Group	$253,400
Warren Surveys	$243,466

These numbers make it apparent that some physicians do very well financially – particularly surgical specialists.

That's a good thing.

Those who are able to meet the challenge of one of the toughest academic obstacle courses in the world should be rewarded. Those who can thrive through three or more years of rigorous training, putting in 80 hour weeks and operating on minimal sleep should be rewarded. And those who are capable of taking a damaged heart and replacing it – or those capable of performing some similar life-saving medical miracle – should be rewarded.

When it is your child or your spouse on the operating table, you don't think about what the physician is earning – you just hope that the doctor is very good at what he or she does. One way to help ensure that capable people enter medicine is to keep the financial rewards high. Based on an a recent personal experience one of us had involving a family member who had been critically injured in a traffic accident, we are glad that good people are attracted to medicine and that they make good money. The proficient doctors – and the great majority of them are proficient – deserve it.

What is important to consider, however, is that someone capable of becoming a good brain surgeon also may be capable of becoming a good lawyer, software pioneer, or stock broker – all areas where the financial rewards can be comparable to, or in some cases much greater than, medicine. So high incomes alone will not be enough to lure bright young people into medicine – nor should money be medicine's main attraction.

In fact, given the conversations we have had with thousands of doctors, money is relatively low on their list of reasons for entering the medical profession.

The traditional lures of medicine have been the unique emotional rewards inherent to the physician/patient relationship, the ability of physicians to freely exercise their judgment, and the opportunity to have a dramatic impact on patients' lives. The first two attractions have been seriously diminished by changes in the way medicine is paid for and administrated. The third attraction – the opportunity to impact lives – remains the one thing that keeps many physicians going. There will come a time, however, when even the ability to help patients is not enough to counterbalance the down side of practicing medicine.

For some physicians, that day has already arrived.

Chapter 6:
In Case Of Emergency...Stay Away From the ER

Patient to an emergency room physician: "Doctor, doctor I broke my arm in two places!"

Emergency physician: "Stay out of those places."

The physician shortage is more than a statistical abstraction – a matter of computer models and numbers, lacking faces or names. The doctor shortage is going to have a real effect on real people. In some cases, the shortage will be a matter of life and death. In fact, in some cases, it already is.

Consider the hospital emergency room. It's the one place you don't want to visit, either for your own sake, or worse, for the sake of an injured child, spouse, parent or friend. It's also the one place hospitals really don't want you to go.

Why? Because most hospitals lose money on the emergency care they provide. The emergency room (ER) – or the emergency *department* (ED), as emergency medicine professionals prefer to call it – is the most expensive setting in which to provide care. For years, the focus of most hospitals has been to steer patients away from the emergency department if at all possible, and to their own private physicians.

But despite the fact that patients don't want to go to the ER and hospitals don't want them there, the volume of visits to hospital emergency departments nationwide has steadily increased in recent years. Consider the graph below:

Emergency Department Visits Nationwide

1997	95 million
2000	108 million
Increase	14%
Most common complaints	Abdominal pain, Chest pain & Fever

Source: Center for Disease Control

The rise in patient volumes can be attributed in part to a growing population. But the real growth engine is tied to economics, government policy and physician supply. Many people visit the ER because they don't have health insurance. A federal law – the Emergency Medical Treatment and Labor Act (EMTALA) - requires hospitals to provide care to anyone who presents themselves at a hospital emergency room. The ER therefore has become the health care safety net for millions of people, though in many cases they are not truly in need of emergency care. Consider the following response to a survey of 716 hospital emergency department managers conducted by

The Schumacher Group, a large national emergency medicine management firm based in Lafayette, Louisiana.

Is your emergency department a major provider of primary care for the indigent/uninsured in your community?

Yes   80%
No   20%

Source: The Schumacher Group, 2005 Survey of Hospital Emergency Department Administration

In addition to the uninsured, the ER also attracts millions of "under-insured" patients.   Mostly, these are Medicaid patients.   As we mentioned earlier, many physicians today are refusing to see Medicaid patients, so many such patients do not have access to a private physician.   Instead, they rely on the emergency room for care.

However, the group that is really driving up volumes in the emergency department is **privately insured** Americans. According to an October, 2003 report by the Center for Studying Health System Change, privately insured patients accounted for most of the 16% rise in hospital emergency department visits between 1996-97 and 2000-01. See the following chart:

Rise in Visits to the Emergency Department
1996-97/2000-01

Types of patients	Increase
Privately insured	24%
Medicare	10%
Uninsured	10%
Medicaid	0%

Source: Center for Studying Health System Change

Why is the number of privately insured patients visiting the ER rising so sharply?   It's not because the ER is suddenly an attractive place to be.   And it's not because privately insured patients are getting into a dramatically higher number of car accidents or falling off of ladders at a greater rate.

It is, however, a matter of **physician access**. Even privately insured patients are finding it more difficult to see private practice physicians, and so they are falling back on the emergency room for care.   Many of them, like many uninsured or under insured patients, are not really in need of emergency care. They really need to see a family physician, a gastroenterologist, a cardiologist, a neurologist or some other type of doctor, but they can't – at least not in the time frame they believe they need to. The chart below indicates that the majority of patients visiting the emergency department are "non-urgent" (i.e., do not have an immediate need to see a doctor.)

Emergency Department Patient Acuity

True emergencies	16%
Urgent	31%
Non-urgent	53%

Source: Center for Disease Control

Who's On Call?

There is a major problem, however, in going to an emergency room with the expectation of seeing a physician – which is that, increasingly, there are not enough physicians willing or able to provide emergency care. This does not mean that there are not physicians working in the emergency room most of the time. The great majority of hospitals generally are able to find emergency medicine physicians or other physicians to be present in the emergency room at all hours. These doctors are trained in diagnosis, stabilizing patients and moving them on to care within the hospital, if need be. But many patients who come to the emergency department – both true emergency patients and non-urgent patients – don't need the types of doctors who are physically present in the ED. What they need are specialists.

For example, someone who has suffered head trauma may need to see a neurosurgeon. Someone who has suffered multiple bone fractures may need an orthopedic surgeon. A child may need a pediatric specialist for any number of reasons. A non-urgent patient with abdominal pains may need to see a gastroenterologist, while another non-urgent patient with a headache may need to see a neurologist. An emergency medicine physician or a family physician working in the emergency department may not have the expertise to perform necessary procedures or make certain diagnoses – in which case, specialists are required.

Hospitals try to arrange for specialists to be "on call" when they are needed in the ER, but it is becoming increasingly difficult to find specialists willing or able to cover the emergency room.

According to The Schumacher Group survey referenced above, over four in ten emergency department administrators say their ERs pose a significant health risk to patients due to lack of specialists willing or able to see emergency patients (see the following.)

Does lack of physician specialty coverage at your emergency department pose a significant health risk to patients?

	2005	2004
Yes	42%	23%
No	58%	69%
N/A	0%	8%

Source: The Schumacher Group, 2005 Hospital Emergency Department Administration Survey

What happens when patients come to the emergency department, but there are no specialists available to see them? By law (EMTALA), the hospital has to "divert" the patient to an ER where there *is* a specialist available. This is a step over half of hospital emergency departments surveyed by The Schumacher Group have had to take in the last 12 months (see below)

In the last 12 months, has lack of physician specialty coverage caused you to divert patients to other hospitals?

	2005	2004
Yes	57%	76%
No	43%	24%

If yes, how often?

	2005	2004
Once every few months	27%	17%
1-2 times a month	25%	21%
3-5 times a month	30%	28%
6 or more times a month	28%	33%
N/A	%	1%

Source: The Schumacher Group 2005 Hospital Emergency Department Administration Survey

Imagine accompanying a loved one who has experienced a traumatic head injury to the ER only to find there is no neurosurgeon available to see him. The nearest facility that does have a neurosurgeon may be on the other side of the city or in an entirely different county.   It's a scary thought, but something like that happens every day and is happening at the majority of hospital ERs throughout the country.

Little wonder that 12% of hospital emergency department managers surveyed by The Schumacher Group indicated they would not go to their own hospital's ER if they were seriously injured – mainly due to lack of specialists available to provide care. (see below)

If you were seriously injured, would you choose to go to your own hospitals ER or would you seek better care elsewhere?

Would go to their own ER	88%
Would go somewhere else	12%

Source: The Schumacher Group 2005 Hospital Emergency Department Administration Survey

Why are specialists unavailable or unwilling to cover the emergency department? Sometimes the problem is simply a matter of supply.   There may not be enough specialists – or any specialists – in the community available to provide emergency room coverage.   This is particularly true in neurosurgery.   Even hospitals in major cities such as Dallas have had difficulty finding neurosurgeons to see emergency patients.

In other cases, communities do have specialists but an increasing number of them are not willing to work in the ER.   Over 30% of hospitals surveyed by The Schumacher Group indicated that they had experienced a drop in the number of specialists willing to provide ER coverage in the last 12 months.   The principal reasons why specialists stopped providing coverage are listed as follows:

Why Specialists Stopped Providing ER Coverage

Discouraged by malpractice concerns	26%
Discouraged by lack of payment for ER services	33%
Specialists recruited away by competition	31%

Source: The Schumacher Group

It is a risky proposition for a neurosurgeon, a cardiologist, an orthopedic surgeon, or other types of surgeons to perform emergency surgery on a patient they have never seen before and about whose medical history they may know nothing.   The chances for a bad outcome under these circumstances are relatively high compared to the controlled conditions surgeons prefer to work under.   Hence, the number of malpractice suits arising from surgery done on emergency patients also is relatively high. Specialists who venture into the ER feel they have targets on their backs and that it is only a matter of time before an unhappy or opportunistic patient will sue them.

Another strong disincentive is the fact that specialists often are poorly reimbursed for the work they perform in the ER, or not reimbursed at all. So the "attractions" of providing ER coverage include:

- Being called into the ER at all hours of the day and night
- Taking the risk of being sued
- Working for little or no pay

In short, the problem is this: A growing number of patients – uninsured, under-insured and fully insured – cannot obtain reasonable access to private practice physicians. Instead, they are going to the ER – and in many cases, they *still* cannot obtain reasonable access to a physician.

This growing challenge – which is becoming an outright crisis in some hospital ERs – is in part a function of the physician shortage. Most doctors have plenty of patients already – they don't need to see the uninsured or the underinsured, and they don't need the headache of working in the ER. We could eliminate these access problems in the ER tomorrow if a national health care plan were implemented and everyone had equal access to private practice physicians.

But if it is hard to access busy physicians today, imagine how difficult it would be to access physicians if everyone was covered by the same national health insurance plan. Giving everyone an equal shot at seeing a physician is only a good idea if there are enough physicians to go around.

We aren't there yet – not even close.

Chapter Seven:
Psychiatry...The Silent Shortage

Psychiatrist to his nurse: "Just say we're very busy. Don't keep saying 'It's a madhouse.'"

A lot of people – many of them physicians – contend that you would have to be crazy to become a doctor today. While we don't necessarily agree (see Chapter 12), it is true that as a group, physicians suffer from a relatively high rate of mental illness.

According to a July 7, 2003 article in *American Medical News,* the newspaper of the American Medical Association, physicians suffer from higher rates of depression and from higher suicide rates than the general public, though they die at much lower rates for virtually every other malady. Female physicians have a higher suicide rate than males, though females in general have a lower suicide rate than males.

And what types of physicians have the highest suicide rate among all doctors? You guessed it – psychiatrists.

Though the rate of depression is particularly high among physicians, depression and other mental illnesses are common throughout the general population, as well. Many of the mentality ill have little to no access to the services of psychiatrists, however. While the doctor shortage is quite apparent at hospital ERs, where patients often flow out into the halls or wait for hours without being seen, it is less apparent in psychiatry. Nevertheless, it is very real. In fact, access to psychiatrists may be more limited than access to any type of medical specialists – but the problem is largely swept under the rug.

That is why we call psychiatry the ***silent shortage.***

Flying under the Radar

If you or a loved one have ever suffered from a serious form of mental illness you are well aware why the need for additional psychiatric services flies under the radar. There is still a stigma attached to mental illness in the United States. Those suffering from depression and other forms of mental illness are reluctant to discuss their problems. Often, they are reluctant to seek treatment.

In addition, mental illnesses generally cannot be addressed through a medical procedure. They can only be cured, or made manageable, through long-term treatment with drugs or therapy. Hospitals and clinics tend to be procedure oriented. Procedures are a "cleaner" form of medicine where you simply perform whatever surgery and testing are necessary and move on to the next patient. If government payers (Medicare/Medicaid) and the private insurance companies pay well for the procedure, great attention is paid to it.   Cardiology procedures and orthopedic surgery procedures usually fall into this highly desirable "profit center" category.

Psychiatry, by contrast, is not a profit center for most hospitals (psychiatric services are not covered by some insurance companies) so such services sometimes are not given a high priority.

But the problem of mental illness is getting too large to ignore.   The federal government, through the Bureau of Health Professions, now lists 1,021 Health Professional Shortage Areas for psychiatry – up from 699 such areas in 1999 (a growth rate of 46%).   It puts the population underserved for psychiatry at over 62 million, up from 47 million in 1999.

A study published in the June 18, 2003 issue of the *Journal of the American Medical Association* puts into perspective the cost and pervasive nature of psychiatric disorders, focusing on depression:

Cost/Scope of Depression

- Annual cost of depression to employers in lost productive time: $44 billion
- Adults who will have major depression at some time in their lives: 16%
- Those seeking professional help who get adequate treatment: 22%

Source: Journal of the American Medical Association (JAMA), June 18, 2003

Ominously, the need for psychiatric services is greatest among two vulnerable populations: children and the poor. Consider:

Child & Adolescent Psychiatry Needs

- About 20% of U.S. children and adolescents (15 million people) ages 7 to 17 have diagnosable psychiatric disorders*

- 9% to 13% of U.S. children and adolescents meet the definition of "serious emotional disturbance."**

- Demand of child and adolescent psychiatrists is projected to increase by 100% between 1995 and 2020, and 19% for general psychiatry***

*Source *Surgeon General*
*   **Center for Mental Health Services*
*   ***Bureau of Health Professions*

While mental health problems are often swept under the rug, there is one area where poor access to mental health services has become apparent – and that is on the streets of most of America's big cities. What many are accustomed to calling the "homeless," are in fact people with acute mental problems who do not have access to adequate mental health services.

Increasingly, these are low income people on Medicaid. Due to budgets cuts at the state level, a lot of Medicaid mental health services are being eliminated, leaving mental health patients with no place to go to find treatment and medication. Without the medications prescribed by psychiatrists, these people usually end up on the street, where they are deemed to be a social problem when in fact they are a medical one. While on the street, many mentally ill people commit a range of crimes, from the petty to the serious. In Texas, for example, 150,000 adults and juveniles who were former patients in the state's public mental health system now are in Texas prisons or jails or are on probation or parole.

Indeed, the Mental Health Association in Texas describes jails and prisons as the "asylums of the new millennium." Many other states are following the same pattern. In the words of David Satcher, MD, former U.S. Surgeon General:

"To a great extent, we are dumping our mental health problems on the streets of America. We are dumping them into our jails and prisons – there's no question about that."

This trend is in part a function of the resources society is prepared to invest in mental health services. When it comes time to cut state budgets, mental health services often are the first item to get the ax. However, physician supply also is playing a growing role. The number of psychiatrists willing or available to see patients – particularly those in the most need of mental health services – is static and will rapidly diminish in the years ahead.

The Oldest Specialty

Psychiatry shares the distinction with cardiovascular surgery as being one of the oldest specialties in medicine – in the sense that physicians in these specialties are on average older than physicians in any other specialty. There are some 41,000 psychiatrists in the United States, according to the American Medical Association. Of these, close to 19,000 (46%) are 55 years old or older, whereas about 30% of all physicians are 55 or older. Close to half of all psychiatrists are therefore at or near retirement age.

In California, the problem is particularly acute. Over 70% of psychiatrists in the Golden State are 50 years old or older and the mental health system is feeling the strain. The closure of a psychiatric facility in the Antelope Valley in May, 2005 due to lack of sufficient psychiatrists is a harbinger of things to come.

Given the shifting attitude toward medicine among older physicians as described in Chapter 4, we expect many of these psychiatrists to retire, find non-clinical jobs, or reduce their patient loads in the next one to three years.

Meanwhile, the total number of physicians training to be psychiatrists has remained static for the last ten years, according to the American Academy of Child & Adolescent Psychiatry. The number of physicians training to be child and adolescent psychiatrists, however, has declined from 712 in 1990 to 657 in 2001, the Academy reports, and the number of child and adolescent psychiatry programs has declined by seven to a total of 113.

These numbers make for some very ominous forecasts. According to the U.S. Bureau of Health Professions, a division of the Department of Health and Human Services, there will be 8,312 child and adolescent psychiatrists in 2020, though 12,624 will be needed to meet demand.

Other numbers contribute to the emerging "perfect storm" in psychiatry. About one third of psychiatrists in active patient care are women, compared to one quarter of all physicians in active patient care. As we discussed in Chapter 3, female physicians work fewer hours per week than male physicians, and so as more women concentrate in certain specialties such as psychiatry, the total workforce in those specialties decreases.

In addition, about one-third of psychiatrists in the United States who are actively involved in patient care are international medical graduates (IMGs), compared to 24% of physicians overall. As we referenced in Chapter 2, the U.S. can no longer rely on a steady influx of IMGs to help fill gaps.

An increasing demand, a static supply, an extraordinarily high percentage of older physicians, women and IMGs...no specialty is subject to as many factors likely to create a physician shortage as is psychiatry.

The results are already being felt. One of the staffing firms within our group of health care staffing companies – Staff Care, Inc. – specializes in filling temporary work assignments for physicians. While temporary physicians are the subject of the next chapter, it is important to note here that the number one need among Staff Care's clients is for psychiatrists.

Many of these clients are government facilities such as prisons, mental hospitals or military/veterans facilities which, increasingly, are charged with providing mental health services to the poor and uninsured. These government facilities are experiencing a great deal of difficulty in finding psychiatrists willing to work on a permanent basis, and so must rely on temporary physicians to fill the gap.

We have found that the temporary physician staffing market predicts the permanent market, and that is being born out in psychiatry. Four to five years ago, Merritt, Hawkins & Associates, which specializes in placing physicians on a permanent basis, had few requests to recruit psychiatrists. Now, psychiatrists are among our top ten most requested searches and rising fast.

For now, access to psychiatric services is severely limited among the poor or the incarcerated, largely due to lack of government funding. A growing part of the equation however, revolves around the fact that while our mental health problems are not going away, our psychiatrists are. It is a problem that is easily swept under the rug – until you, your child, or your parent experiences a mental health problem.

Then, it's a crisis.

Chapter 8:
Have Stethoscope/Will Travel

"In traveling, a man must bring knowledge with him, if he would bring knowledge home." – Samuel Johnson

Temporary workers ("temps") generally are adept at filing, typing and other clerical tasks. Employers expect punctuality and efficiency from temps, but rarely do they expect temps to be brain surgeons.

Unless, of course, we are talking about **temporary physicians**, which in this chapter, we are. An increasing number of doctors work as temps – only in medicine temporary physicians are known *"locum tenens"* physicians. Locum tenens is a Latin term for "one holding a place."

Locum tenens physicians are becoming the "Lone Rangers" of health care. They ride into towns needing additional medical services, take on the "bad guys" (flu, lacerations, brain contusions, whatever) and then ride away again, without ever asking for a "thank you" (though they are paid a daily rate.)

Sometimes hospitals and medical groups use locum tenens physicians because a temporary need has arisen in their communities. For example, a radiologist may be going on vacation for a month, so a locum tenens radiologist is brought in to provide services until the permanent doctor comes back. Or a community may be undergoing a heavy flu season and need an extra family physician to handle patient overflow.

More typically, however, hospitals and medical groups are turning to locum tenens doctors to plug in gaps in their medical staffs. While they are looking for a permanent gastroenterologist, radiologist or psychiatrist, they keep the ship afloat with temporary, locum tenens doctors.

Going Mobile

This phenomenon is quite common throughout healthcare and is particularly prevalent in nursing. Though patients may not realize it, many of the nurses in the hospital they encounter are not employed by the hospital. Instead, they are "contract" or "per diem" nurses the hospital is using to maintain services while (hopefully) building their permanent nurse staff. Some hospitals, however, have become "temp dependent" and feel compelled to rely on temporary nurses indefinitely because they cannot find enough permanent nurses to fill openings.

These nurses generally work through agencies which schedule them at various hospitals on temporary assignments that typically range from one day to three months. Temporary nurses and other health care workers generally are paid more per hour than permanent workers, while often still receiving benefits such as health insurance or malpractice insurance. Some hospital staffs use few contract nurses, but at other hospitals, one-third of the nursing staff or more may be comprised of temporary nurses. Many radiologic technologists – the people who operate x-ray machines, CTs, MRI scanners and other diagnostic equipment – also are working on a temporary basis, as are certified registered nurse anesthetists (CRNAs) and other allied health professionals.

In the last ten years, the work force model in health care has shifted from a relatively stable one to an increasingly mobile one, in which a growing group of traveling health professionals circulate around the country plugging a leak here while another leak springs up there. The growth of the locum tenens industry clearly illustrates this trend.

Just six or seven years ago the locum tenens industry was a somewhat low profile segment of the health care staffing market. Locum tenens physicians were for the most part older doctors in semi retirement mode who would work a few months of the year on a temporary basis to supplement their incomes. Consider how the industry has grown in the last seven years, however:

Spending On Locum Tenens Staffing Services

2002	*2001*	*2000*	*1999*	*1998*	*1997*
$2.8 bil	$1.93 bil	$1.25 bil	$899 mil	$684 mil	$479 mil

Source: Staff Care, Inc. 2003 Review of Temporary Healthcare Staffing Trends/Incentives

Not only have hospitals and other health care providers been spending more on locum tenens services in an attempt to maintain staffing levels, but more physicians have elected to work as "temps."

Number Of Physicians Working Locum Tenens

1997	15,000
2003	29,000

Source: Staff Care, Inc., 2003 Review of Temporary Healthcare Staffing Trends

More physicians are attracted to the locum tenens style of practice because of the relative freedom it affords them from many of the "hassle factors" of medicine we discussed in Chapters 2 and 3. Locum tenens doctors don't have to deal with third party payors such as Medicare or managed care plans. They are paid on a per diem basis by the staffing agencies through which they work, such as our company, Staff Care, Inc.

Staffing firms provide them with malpractice coverage, as well as a range of assignments that may take them from San Francisco one month to Frisco, Texas the next. Locum tenens doctors spend most of their time with patients, and relatively little time with reimbursement related paperwork or medical politics. While they may not make as much money as a physician in traditional practice, the money is still quite good and there is no practice overhead or administrative issues to worry about.

Given these attractions and the increasing use of locum tenens physicians, a different type of physician is being attracted to temporary practice. No longer is locum tenens the province of older physicians in semi-retirement. An increasing number are younger physicians just out of residency who are choosing to work on a temporary basis.

% of Temporary Physicians 1 To 2 Years Out of Residency

2003	13%
2001	11%
2000	7%

Source: Staff Care, Inc. 2003 Review of Temporary Healthcare Staffing Trends

Younger physicians find that working locum tenens gives them the opportunity to "test drive" different practice locations and different practice styles. By the time they have completed a few assignments, they may know what medical practice is like in a rural community that supports a 30-bed hospital and in an urban community that supports a 300-bed hospital. It also is a good way for young physicians to enjoy more family time, as they can work for a few months, and then spend a few months at home. Working locum tenens, younger physicians don't have to invest the enormous amount of time it takes running a practice or being on the staff of a hospital or medical group.

Originally, locum tenens was intended to bring some staffing relief to mostly isolated, rurally based hospitals. The focus generally was on primary care, but that, too, has shifted. The graph below indicates the specialties in greatest demand among those using locum tenens physicians, and indicates the number of locum tenens opportunities available for physicians in each specialty:

Top Ten Locum Tenens Specialties, 2002

Specialty	% Total demand	Opportunities per physician
Psychiatry	17%	3.60
Radiology	14%	2.94
Family practice	11%	1.54
Anesthesiology	9%	2.61
Internal medicine	7%	1.59
Child psychiatry	3%	7.77
Emergency medicine	3%	2.07
Cardiology	2%	2.43
Orthopedic surgery	2%	4.25
Gastroenterology	2%	3.09

Source: Staff Care, 2003 Market Analysis and Executive Summary, Temporary Healthcare Staffing

While family practice and internal medicine are prominent on the list, the majority of demand in locum tenens is coming from psychiatry, radiology, anesthesiology and other medical specialties. The medical facilities that use these physicians breakout into three categories, as follows:

Private facilities	VA, Military, Indian Health	Correctional
65%	15%	20%

Source: Staff Care, Inc.

While the use of locum tenens physicians is proportionately higher at facilities that sometimes have limited appeal to physicians, such as veterans' hospitals or correctional facilities, a large number of private hospitals that are relatively attractive to physicians also have come to rely on temporary doctors.

You would be hard pressed to find any profession outside of health care where job opportunities are so abundant that tens of thousands of workers can roam the country picking those locations that interest them and earning a higher hourly wage than permanent workers are afforded.

Locum tenens physicians provide a valuable service to communities and facilities in need of more physicians. This growing style of practice is a way for older physicians to see fewer patients while still earning a decent living. It also is a way for younger physicians to balance work and lifestyle needs. But as more physicians embrace a temporary style of practice, the number of hours they work on average decreases. When two physicians complete training, and both are working only half the year, only one "full time equivalent physician" has in fact entered the work force.

We have made the point before, but it is worth repeating. *How many* physicians there are is just one part of the equation. *How they practice* also must be considered. As more physicians and other health professionals are attracted by the benefits of working on a temporary basis, the total number of "full-time equivalent" (FTE) workers decreases.

It's one more reason why we need to train more doctors.

Chapter Nine:
Hospitals And Physicians...Can't We All Just Get Along?

Doctor: "We need to get these people to a hospital."

Nurse: "What is it?"

Doctor: "A big building with a lot of doctors, but that's not important now."

As an article in the March 3, 2004 edition of *The Wall Street Journal* points out, hospitals in the 19th Century had a rather unfortunate nickname from a public relations point of view. They were referred to as "gateways to death."

Hospitals originally were private, charitable institutions set up for the "deserving poor." If you had money, you didn't go there. Instead, physicians came to your home, routinely performing deliveries and even surgery on the patient's furniture. As private institutions, hospitals reserved the right to deny care to anyone. The chronically sick, such as cancer patients, often were turned away, as were the "morally unworthy," such as alcoholics or prostitutes.

As the *Wall Street Journal* piece further points out, some hospitals required a letter of recommendation from an upstanding citizen before they would admit a patient. Many would not admit minorities. As late as 1922, almost a quarter of all general hospitals in the U.S. served white people only.

In addition to being unsanitary, hospitals had few treatments to offer and almost no cures. Hospitals were places that simply tried to keep patients alive through a serious illness or injury, providing a warm bed, milk, meat, and potatoes. In the 1870s and 1880s, "the average stay at a private hospital was two to three months. Some patients stayed for years," according to the *WSJ*. You didn't get much, but then it didn't cost much, either. In 1880, the cost of keeping a patient in New York's St. John's hospital for a day was 80 cents, or $14 in today's money. One of the principal line items was the house physician's salary – $300 a year in the case of St. John's. By contrast, a hospital in 2004 will pay over $1,000 *a day* for a locum tenens physician to see patients.

So while hospital stays were relatively cheap, you often got what you paid for, which was very little in the way of useful treatment.

It's Getting Better All the Time

For those pessimists who think life is only getting worse, consider American hospitals today. If you have a serious health problem – if you need brain surgery, a new heart, or if you need an outright miracle, such as the separation of conjoined twins – there is no better place to be. The world knows this, and increasingly people from other countries are beating a path to our door for advanced health care. This is yet another reason why we should be training more physicians. We need doctors to not only treat our own population, but the growing number of people worldwide who seek American medical expertise.

Over the last 100 years, hospitals have become the innovators and purchasers of expanding medical technology. The development of specialized diagnostic, surgical and drug technology has gone hand in hand with the increasingly close relationship between hospitals and physicians. The nation's 700 teaching hospitals are where physicians get their advanced training. They learn to be doctors in the hospital environment, using all the personnel and technological resources hospitals bring to bear. Often, the patients they see and the procedures they perform are conducted in the hospital.

In the past, this relationship has been mostly symbiotic. Hospitals provided physicians with training and with the tools, the setting, and the personnel to do their jobs. Physicians provided hospitals with both their expertise and with patients. Through referrals, physicians traditionally have been the primary source of patients for hospitals. Without an active group of loyal "admitters" on the staff sending patients their way, hospitals lack the "customers" they need to remain financially viable.

Ideally, the glue that cements the physician/hospital relationship is patient welfare. The mission of physicians is to serve their patients. The mission of hospitals is to serve their communities, which are comprised of patients and potential patients. Patient welfare is the fundamental value or goal that should foster physician/hospital cooperation.

Open Warfare

Lately, however, that glue has been coming apart. The conflict between hospitals and physicians has been simmering for decades, and lately it has broken out into outright warfare. Increasingly, hospitals and physicians are not working in tandem but are in overt competition with one another. The most visible sign of this is the hundred-plus "specialty hospitals" that have arisen around the country in the last several years. These hospitals usually specialize in the treatment of one area, such as the heart or the musculoskeletal system. That is why hospital administrators sometimes ruefully refer to the rise of specialty hospitals as the "invasion of the body part snatchers." In most cases, specialty hospitals are owned by physicians.

Specialty hospitals make an effort to offer "all the amenities of home" – comfortable beds, good food, designer coffees, etc., and they often attract more affluent patients than do traditional acute care hospitals. They usually are in direct competition with acute care hospitals which often are not able to provide such a wide range of amenities and which are obliged to treat all kinds of patients. It is yet to be seen whether the moratorium placed by Congress on the building of these hospitals will be extended.

In addition to specialty hospitals, there are some 3,000 to 4,000 physician-owned surgery centers and diagnostic centers across the country that provide treatment or diagnosis that in the past were almost always performed in the hospital. These centers provide outpatient procedures that do not require overnight stays or much patient monitoring. They also feature the amenities of home (latte with that shoulder surgery, sir?) Surgery or diagnosis is performed and within an hour or two the patient leaves the surgery center under his or her own power. Physicians also now perform many surgeries or diagnostic procedures in their offices.

Due to improvements in medical technology, the amount of outpatient or ambulatory surgery has exploded in recent years, as the graph below illustrates:

Growth of Outpatient Surgery in the U.S.

Outpatient surgeries, 1980	15% of all surgeries
Outpatient surgeries, 2000	70% of all surgeries
# of outpatient surgeries, 1990	2.3 million
# of outpatient surgeries, 2000	6.7 million

Source: American Medical News, April 15, 2002

These procedures often are lucrative in part because they do not entail expensive overnight stays, and both hospitals and physicians are vying for this type of work. Physicians appear to be winning the battle, however, as the figures below attest:

Ambulatory Surgery Volumes Compound Annual Growth Rates 1981-2007

13.8%	13.4%	8.1%
Free standing clinic (physician owned)	Physician Office	Hospital

When physicians defect from traditional acute care hospitals to their own specialty hospitals, the economic consequences for the traditional facilities are severe.   The chart below indicates the average revenue physicians in various specialties generate per year for the hospitals with which they are affiliated:

Inpatient/Outpatient Average Net Revenue Generated for Hospitals by Physicians

Specialty	*Revenue*
Orthopedic Surgery	$2,992,022
Cardiology (non-inv.)	$2,646,039
Cardiovascular (inv.)	$2,490,748
General Surgery	$2,446,987
Neuro Surgery	$2,406,275
Internal Medicine	$2,100,124
Family Practice	$2,000,329
OB/GYN	$1,903,919
Hematology/ Oncology	$1,802,749
Pulmonology	$1,781,578
Gastroenterology	$1,735,338
Psychiatry	$1,332,948
Urology	$1,317,415
Nephrology	$1,121,000
Neurology	$924,798
Pediatrics	$860,600

Source: Merritt, Hawkins & Associates 2004 Survey of Physician Inpatient/Outpatient Revenue

On average, a physician will put $1.85 million a year into his or her affiliated hospital through patient referrals and admissions.   Hospitals hate to see physician defections and argue that specialty hospitals and physician-run surgery centers siphon away the lucrative procedures and high paying patients and leave hospitals as the social safety net to take care of indigent or poor paying patients.

Poor patients go to the "regular" hospital.   More affluent patients no longer have physicians come to their homes, but they get all the comforts of home at a specialty hospital.

Sounds like we have come full circle, doesn't it?

Origins of the Conflict

Why have physicians and hospitals become increasingly adversarial, how can this problem be addressed, and where does the supply of physicians fit into the picture?

Most misunderstandings arise from differing perspectives, and that is the case in the conflict between physicians and hospitals. The people who run hospitals – "health care administrators" – often have a different outlook on things than physicians. Physicians typically are:

- Clinically/scientifically oriented
- Soloists at heart
- Have "circled the wagons"
- Are suspicious of the administrative role in medicine

Administrators, by contrast, generally are:

- Accustomed to a "top-down" management hierarchy
- Team-oriented
- Responsible for the "bottom line"

To physicians, patient care is paramount, and, as soloists and highly trained scientists, they expect to have the final word regarding how patient care is conducted. Administrators must look at the bigger picture of how resources are allocated and what is best in the long run for the hospital as an institution and the community it serves. Used to the "chain of command" that is prevalent in business, administrators expect that everyone in the hierarchy will follow the plan. For reasons previously stated, physicians have become increasingly sensitive to any challenge to their autonomy, and resist when they feel they are being dictated to. Managing physicians, a common expression goes, is like "herding cats." That is one reason why "managed care" – the attempt to direct how physicians practice – did not succeed.

The result is that many physicians want to do things their way – at their own hospitals, surgery centers or offices. This can be more lucrative for them, and the movement toward physician hospital ownership is certainly in part driven by financial considerations. What physicians also are seeking, however, is more efficiency and more control. Consider the remarks of a family physician explaining why she refers patients to ambulatory surgery centers when she can, rather than to a hospital:

"It's not that (referring physicians) prefer ambulatory surgery centers. But we do prefer a quick treatment and an effective treatment in a safe environment."

Source: *American Medical News, April 15, 2002*

In the past, hospitals have tried to build physician support and loyalty by involving doctors in hospital management or giving them more influence by placing them on the hospital's board of directors. But this method may have a limited influence on physician loyalty, as the following remarks by a physician attest:

"I don't think many of us feel the immediacy of what the hospital is planning over the next five year or how many physicians are on the Board (of Directors .) But we do feel an immediacy toward whether or not the stat results from the lab get back in two hours or eight hours."

Source: Health Care Advisory Board Study

Nor do physicians require much help from hospitals in marketing their practices. These days, there are plenty of patients to go around.

The key for hospitals, then, is to offer physicians what they really want, which is:

- Easy access to the hospital – location of hospital and parking are top concerns
- Efficiency – easy access for patients, quick turnaround of diagnostics, easy access to patient data
- Competent, well trained nurses
- Competent, well trained fellow physicians
- Up-to-date equipment

In turn, what hospitals would like to see from physicians is a greater awareness of the need to provide care appropriately, but cost-effectively, and a greater acknowledgement of the long-term role hospitals play in serving the health needs of all members of the community.

Again, the common denominator is patient welfare. It should and can be the unifying factor that ensures a more symbiotic relationship between hospitals and physicians.

The Role of Physician Supply

The number of places where health care services are being performed is expanding, but the number of physicians is not. Traditional hospitals now sometimes have to compete against specialty hospitals in physician recruitment, or against medical groups that are competing directly against the hospital. A community may not necessarily need two more vascular surgeons – one for the specialty hospital and one for the traditional hospital – but that is what it may get.

Meanwhile, other communities that do need a vascular surgeon may have to do without. That is not the ideal method of physician distribution, but in today's recruiting market, the fact is that the physician you gain may be the physician another community loses.

With physician supply in its current state, you sometimes have to rob Peter to pay Paul. This would seem to create a favorable market for physician recruiters like ourselves, but it puts stress on the system and is not in the best interests of patient care. And even for physician recruiters, the dearth of doctors can be more a curse than a blessing. Our product is physicians and we need to deliver, but in some cases today certain types of doctors simply may not be available. It would be an advantage from our perspective if more potential recruits were coming out of residency each year. We certainly would not like to see a surplus of physicians, but the well today is too dry for our comfort.

The conflict between physicians and hospitals and the strain on all parties would be eased if there were more physicians to go around. More doctors would create greater access for both those parties recruiting physicians and for those patients who need physicians – whether they are affluent patients or the un or under-insured.

When resources become too scarce, they are fought over. When they become too abundant, they are undervalued.

What we need is a happy medium.

Chapter 10:
The Vanishing Country Doctor

"Don't live in a town with no doctors." – Jewish Proverb

Some things today are just plain hard to find. Good taste on television. Honest baseball records. A needle in a haystack. Country doctors.

Country doctors have been in short supply for decades. Even those physician supply experts who thought the U.S. had too many doctors always acknowledged that we had too few willing to practice in rural areas. Rather than an outright shortage of physicians, however, they argued that we had a maldistribution. A lot of doctors practiced in the city, but not many practiced in the country. It was hoped that the surplus of doctors in the city would find its way out into the country. Instead, the dearth of doctors in the country seems to have found its way into the city.

Meanwhile, the number of physicians in rural America is ebbing, while demand is likely to rise faster in the country than anywhere else. The National Rural Health Association (as referenced in the March 8, 2004 issue of the *Nashville Business Journal*) indicates that over 20% of the U.S. population resides in rural areas, but less than 11% of the nation's physicians practice there. Meanwhile, 16% of the rural population lives in poverty, compared to 13% of the total population, while 18% are elderly, compared to 15% of the total population. Generally, the poor and the elderly require more medical services than the affluent and the young.

We mentioned previously that there are over 2,500 federally designated Health Care Professional Shortage Areas (HPSAs) in the U.S. Of these, the great majority are in rural areas. An estimated 35 million Americans live in HPSAs where 16,000 more physicians would be needed to alleviate the physician shortage, according to a report prepared by the Department of Sociology at DePaul University cited in the March 16, 2004 edition of *Modern Physician*. Over half a million Americans live in counties where there are no practicing physicians at all.

Rural physicians also are older than urban ones. 15% of rural physicians are over 65, compared to 13% of all physicians. Who will replace these older doctors when they retire or die?

Therein lies the rub. Only some 6% of final year medical residents surveyed by Merritt, Hawkins & Associates indicated they wanted to practice in small towns. It is very difficult to attract physicians to rural practice these days for several reasons.

First, the great majority of doctors train in large, urban teaching hospitals. They are accustomed to having a lot of technical resources at their disposal and many specialists on-site for back up. Many are leery of being thrown out on their own in rural America. In addition, the hours and practice style can be more demanding, particularly because they have to be "on call" more often than urban doctors And most doctors want the same things from a community that other professionals want – movie theaters, restaurants, opera companies, professional sports and other amenities that the country sometimes can't offer.

Perhaps the biggest impediment to attracting physicians to rural areas (alluded to in Chapter 2), is what is known as "trailing spouse syndrome." In the "old days" physicians were predominantly male and they were the sole breadwinners in the family. Today, many physician spouses – both male and female – also are professionals such as lawyers, accountants, computer programmers, writers, architects, etc. While there is plenty of work in smaller communities for physicians, there often is little work for their spouses. Attracting a physician to a community really means attracting his or her whole family. No work for the spouse – or inadequate amenities for the children, such as a top ranked gymnastics program or a renowned piano instructor – can be a recruitment deal killer, and often is.

For this reason alone, doctors are likely to be in short supply in rural America for the foreseeable future. This is unfortunate, since "country medicine" can be a very satisfying style of practice and since the need is so great.

For that reason, one of our companies (Staff Care, Inc.) has chosen to highlight the accomplishments of rural practitioners and to promote rural medical practice through the *"Country Doctor of the Year Award."* Every year, Staff Care receives hundreds of nominations for this award submitted by health care professionals or average citizens of small towns wishing to honor their country doctors. Winners of the award have been profiled nationally in media outlets that include *People* magazine, *Parade, USA Today* and *"The Today Show."*

These are all outstanding medical practitioners who exemplify the spirit, skill and dedication of the country doctor, and we would like to introduce them to you.

Meet Ten Great Country Doctors.

In chronological order, the Country Doctors of the Year are:

John Harlan Haynes, Country Doctor of the Year, 1992
Vivian, Louisiana. Population 4156

Described by his patients as "a cross between Daniel Boone and Marcus Welby," Dr. Haynes has practiced in this rural community for over 35 years, single-handedly keeping the hospital open. Renowned for his diagnostic ability, Dr. Haynes is known as a friend and a lifesaver throughout eastern Louisiana.

Claire Louise Caudill, Country Doctor of the Year, 1993
Morehead, Kentucky. Population 8357

Known as "The Mother of Rowan County," Dr. Caudill, now deceased, delivered over 8,000 babies in her 50-year career and was noted for her house calls to people in the "hollers" of rural Kentucky. Dr. Caudill is a legend in her region of the state. Both a play and a book have been written about her, and St. Claire Hospital in Morehead was named in her honor.

William Hill, Country Doctor of the Year, 1994
Carrolton, Alabama. Population 1170

"Dr. William" served as a solo physician in Carrolton for over 50 years, carrying on a family tradition. Hill family physicians have served Carrolton continuously since before the Civil War.

Elton D. Lehman, Country Doctor of the Year, 1996 (no candidate selected in 1995)
Mount Eaton, Ohio. Population 250

For 34 years, Dr. Lehman brought modern medicine to the Amish community of Stark County, while also serving as the town's mayor. Dr. Lehman helped design, fund, and build a free-standing birthing center for Amish women as a safer alternative to home delivery.   The center features a hitching post for horses and buggies and gas rather than electric lamps to help Amish patients feel more comfortable.

Paul F. Maddox, Country Doctor of the Year, 1998 (no candidate selected in 1997)
Campton, Kentucky. Population 525

Dr. Maddox treated over 1.5 million patients during his 47-year career.   During much of that time he was the only physician serving an entire county, treating many patients free of charge. Dr. Maddox kept his clinic open 24 hours a day, 365-days a year for two decades – while serving as the town's mayor. He continues to practice at age 74 even after being diagnosed with cancer, scheduling patients around daily chemotherapy.

Howard Clark, Country Doctor of the Year, 1999
Morton, Mississippi. Population 4,000

At age 73, Dr. Clark still works more than 90 hours a week, covering his clinic practice, the hospital emergency room, and the nursing home and making house calls. He was largely responsible for reopening the county hospital and once covered the emergency room for 23 consecutive days – at no charge. Dr. Clark routinely treats patients regardless of their ability to pay and did not miss a local high school football game for which he was the team doctor from 1956 to 2000.

Kamlesh Gosai, Country Doctor of the Year, 2001 (no candidate selected in 2000)
Bentleyville, Pennsylvania. Population 2,700

Prior to recruiting Dr. Gosai, Bentleyville had tried to recruit a physician without success, though they were offering a new building with rent-free office space and financial incentives. When Dr. Gosai set up shop in 1988, he declined all incentives and simply got to work. He now sees more than 300 patients a week regardless of their ability to pay and he has recruited six other doctors. Residents credit him for saving a dying town by restoring health care services, developing a medical laboratory with MRI, and spearheading the creation of an industrial park. In his "spare time" he visits 21 nursing and personal care homes and makes hospital rounds.

James Blume, Country Doctor of the Year, 2002
Forest Hill, West Virginia. Population 75

Diagnosed with colon cancer in 2001, Dr. Blume ignored the effects of chemotherapy and kept treating patients at his small town clinic. At times he was so weak he leaned against walls for support while working. Yet he also broke ground on an urgent care center 14 miles away and volunteered to deliver four sermons a week after a nearby church lost its pastor. Despite a malpractice crisis that drove many physicians away from West Virginia, Dr. Blume chose to sell a bit of property in order to cover insurance costs so he could continue providing care to residents of Forest Hill.

Charles Boyette, Country Doctor of the Year, 2003
Belhaven, North Carolina

When Hurricane Isabel descended on North Carolina, many people fled. Dr. Boyette gathered up medical supplies and prepared his home to serve as a temporary emergency room, treating a variety of injuries and a heart attack. This is illustrative of Dr. Boyette's commitment to Belhaven, where he rescued the local hospital from bankruptcy, launched a foundation providing financial aid to over 100 community college students and served as major. And he still makes house calls.

Kenneth Paul Mauterer, Jr., Country Doctor of the Year, 2004
Olla, Louisiana

Doctor "Kenny Paul" as he is known to the residents of Olla is a true home-grown hero. The community helped put Dr. Mauterer through medical school and he returned the favor by practicing in his home town for the last 30 years, single handedly keeping the local hospital open for much of that time.

Vanishing Legends

What most of these legendary doctors have in common, in addition to their extraordinarily high commitment to their patients, is that they are 70 years old or older, already retired, or deceased. Only doctors Blume, Gosai and Mauterer are likely to provide medical care to their communities for the long-term.

Who will replace these great country doctors when they are gone? The answer to that question remains very uncertain.

Chapter 11:
The Supporting Cast

Question: How many doctors does it take to change a light bulb?

Answer: One, but the light bulb has to revolve around him.

It used to be that the doctor and the nurse were the Batman and Robin of the medical team. That is no longer the case today. By the time a patient is diagnosed and has a routine surgery performed, he is likely to be treated by a variety of physicians and a multi-member team of "allied health care professionals," including

- A radiologic technologist: to take the x-rays, CT, MRI or other images required
- A certified registered nurse anesthetist (CRNA): to assist in providing anesthesia
- A physician assistant (PA) or nurse practitioner (NP): to assist with the surgery
- A laboratory technologist (LT) to process lab tests
- A physical therapist (PT): to assist with post-operative recovery
- A pharmacist: to fill drug prescriptions

Allied professionals are all those people who provide medical care – including nurses – who are not physicians. There are millions of these professionals throughout the U.S. but, like physicians, they generally are in short supply. The following graph illustrates hospital vacancy rates for allied health care professionals.

Hospital Vacancy Rates

Pharmacists	21%
Radiologic technologists	18%
Laboratory technologists	12%
Registered nurses	11%

Source: American Hospital Association

It is difficult to fill these positions not only because workers are in short supply but because turnover rates among health care workers are relatively high (see below.)

Annual Turnover Rates for Allied Health Professionals

Nurses	15.5%
Occupational therapists	14.9%
Respiratory therapists	14.2%
Speech/language therapists	14.0%
Physical therapists	13.5%
Radiologic technologists	12.1%
Pharmacits	12.0%
Laboratory technicians	10.7%

Source: Bernard Hodes Group, as referenced in Modern Healthcare, 12/2/03

The national shortage of nurses has been well documented and most people who read the newspapers are probably aware by now that the U.S. has too few nurses. Indeed, for the first time, registered nurses top the U.S. Bureau of Labor Statistics' list of occupations with the largest projected 10-year job growth. The bureau's last projections, as reported in the February 23, 2004 edition of *Modern Healthcare* magazine, put the demand for registered nurses at 2.9 million in 2012. The total number of RN job openings between now and 2012 will be 1.1 million, the Bureau projects.

Though the number of people seeking to enter nurse training programs has increased in the last three years, the Bureau points out that there are too few teachers, classrooms or clinical sites to handle all qualified applicants. In short, we can't train people fast enough to become nurses, even though interest in the profession has increased. Some forecasters predict that there will be about 500,000 too few nurses in the U.S. in the next decade.

This is bad news for patients, because studies have shown a direct relationship between the number of nurses per patient and mortality rates in hospitals. For example, a study conducted by the University of Pennsylvania found that patients at hospitals with a high number of patients-to-nurses (twelve patients per nurse) had a 31% greater risk of dying than patients at hospitals with a low number of patients-to-nurses (eight patients per nurse.) The Joint Commission on Accreditation of Healthcare Organizations, as referenced in the March 30, 2004 edition of the *Kansas City Star,* indicates that nurse shortages are a factor in about one-fourth of patient injuries or deaths at hospitals. The same newspaper story references a Harvard and Vanderbilt university study indicating that preventable deaths and patient complication rates were up to nine times higher in hospitals where the most care was given by licensed practical nurses and aides, not by registered nurses.

It is for this reason that California passed a law mandating that hospitals maintain a certain level of nurses per patient. Other states are expected to follow suit soon.

While such "mandatory nurse staffing laws" may have patient welfare in mind, they are out of tune with the realities of nurse staffing. Some hospitals simply cannot find the nurses they need. These hospitals would like to maintain a higher ratio of nurses to patients, but as a practical matter they are not always able to do so. In some instances, hospitals that cannot find the requisite number of nurses must shut down hospital beds, or even entire wings. This includes shutting down beds in the emergency department.

As we have noted earlier, hospital visits – and visits to the ER, in particular – are steadily increasing. This is an inopportune time to decrease access to medical services, but staffing deficiencies combined with mandatory nurse-to-patient ratios are making it inevitable.

In the past, foreign-born nurses have acted as a supplement to the workforce when U.S. nurses have been in short supply. As with physicians, however, current immigration law does not favor the employment of foreign born nurses. The principal problem is that there is no tenable temporary work visa category for nurses. Dozens of foreign born professionals of all kinds can work in the U.S. on temporary work visas, but for the most part nurses cannot.

Carl Shusterman, a prominent Los Angeles immigration attorney who has testified before Congress on nurse immigration issues, points out that foreign born fashion models can obtain temporary work visas, but the great majority of nurses cannot – an interesting comment on our national priorities (anyone interested in a comprehensive review of this topic should check out Mr. Shusterman's web site at www.shusterman.com.)

Since we are unable to train the nurses we need domestically and since the supply of foreign nurses is significantly limited by immigration law, we can expect the nurse shortage to be with us for some time.

It's Not Just RNs

Though the nurse shortage gets most of the ink when it comes to health care staffing issues, nurses aren't the only members of the health care team in short supply. The following graph illustrates the jobs hospitals find are the hardest to fill:

Jobs Hospitals Are Struggling To Fill

Registered nurse	84%
Radiology/nuclear imaging	71%
Pharmacy	46%
Lab/medical technology	27%

Source: American Hospital Assn. Survey, Modern Healthcare, Dec. 22, 2003

While nurses are tough to find, over two-thirds of hospitals are struggling to recruit radiologic technologists – the people who operate diagnostic equipment such as x-rays, CT, MRI, nuclear imaging, PET, ultrasound, mammography, and all the other diagnostic imaging "modalities."

We have previously observed that in health care today, "imaging is everything." Almost nothing can be done by way of diagnosis or surgery today without a picture, and it is the "rad techs" who take the hundreds of millions of diagnostic images captured each year. In fact, the "face" of the hospital today as often as not is the rad tech, not the nurse. It is the tech who the patient sees when he or she comes into the hospital for a CT scan or for an ultrasound – not the nurse. Often, a patient will judge his or her hospital experience based on how long it took for the imaging process to be completed and on how courteously they were treated by the tech. For this reason – and because hospitals make a tremendous amount of money from diagnostic imaging – technologists have become very important members of the health care team.

However, the supply trend in radiologic technology is not much brighter than it is in nursing. There are some 300,000 imaging technologists practicing various imaging modalities today. According to the national health care consulting firm Solucient, demand for imaging services will increase 67% between 2002 and 2007. We won't be able to train techs fast enough to meet this demand. The American Society of Radiologic Technology (ASRT), the national professional association for imaging technologists, projects that the supply of technologists will fall 30% short of what the Bureau of Labor Statistics says will be needed by 2010.

As with nursing, more people are interested in becoming technologists, but the educational resources are not there to train them. About 80% of all training programs surveyed by the ASRT in 2003 were at full capacity and had to turn away 23,550 qualified applicants, mostly due to insufficient faculty and space. So the technologist shortage also is one that will not be resolved any time soon.

Pharmacy is another area where shortages are likely to be protracted. We referenced earlier the boom in prescription drugs, which is an inescapable fact of life for those of us who have to deal with email spam. Prescription drugs have gone commercial and are being marketed directly to the consumer, through television, print, and most intrusively through the Internet. The number of drugs available and their enhanced effectiveness has dramatically increased the use of pharmacology-based therapies and treatments. Consider the graph below:

Increasing Number of Prescription Drugs

# of prescription drugs, 1973	1,500
# of prescription drugs, 2003	9,000

Source: Trustee magazine, an American Hospital Association publication, February, 2003.

America's appetite for prescription drugs is likely to grow even faster in coming years, thanks to the new Medicare reform bill which offers senior citizens a prescription drug benefit.   Someone is going to have to fill the 4 billion plus (and rising) prescriptions that are being written each year – someone who is well trained in the increasingly complex science of pharmacology.   Both the retail sector (i.e., drug stores) and the clinical sector (i.e., hospitals and medical groups) are clamoring for the services of pharmacists.   Since drug stores usually can pay more, they often are more successful in their recruiting efforts, leaving hospitals and other health care providers short handed.

Both drug stores and hospitals have raised pay levels for pharmacists in an attempt to recruit them.   This has lured many faculty members at pharmacy training programs into the non-academic workforce.   The 80 or so U.S. pharmacy schools will have a difficult time producing the pharmacists we are going to need due to an insufficient number of teachers.   Pharmacy therefore is another area where shortages will be the norm for the foreseeable future.

A Little Sunshine, Please

Shortages of health care workers – physicians and allied professionals – are pervasive throughout the U.S., but not everything is gloom and doom.

For example, the number of physician assistants (PAs) has doubled in the last 10 years, from about 25,000 to 50,000, as reported by the American Academy of Physician Assistants (AAPA) in the December 4, 2003 online issue of *Modern Physician*.   As the name implies, physician assistants are health professionals who support doctors and generally must be supervised by them.   You may have been seen by a PA yourself, either at the doctor's office when you came in for a flu prescription or in the operating room when a PA may have prepped you for surgery.

PAs and advanced practice nurses (NPs) can do many of the things physicians do, including prescribe drugs.   Physicians often employ them to handle patients with a low level of acuity – colds and headaches.   They also can assist in surgery and with helping patients follow their treatment plans.   Like doctors, PAs have certain areas of specialization (see below).

Physician Assistants/Areas of Specialization

Family practice	16,391
Emergency medicine	5,923
General internal medicine	4,373
Orthopedic surgery	3,189
General pediatrics	1,639
OB/GYN	1,482
Occupational medicine	1,438
Cardiovascular surgery	1,410
Cardiology	1,412
General surgery	1,017
Pediatric subspecialties	755

Source: American Academy of Physician Assistants, Modern Physician, 12/4/03

The AAPA reports that PAs saw 192 million patient visits and prescribed 236 million medications in 2003 – numbers that indicate PAs are having a significant effect on patient care.

Both PAs and NPs are to some extent reducing the need for primary care physicians, defined again as family physicians, general internal medicine practitioners and pediatricians. They are having less of an effect reducing the need for specialists, however. While a surgical PA or NP can help prepare a patient for surgery or assist in the patient's post-operative treatment, it is the surgeon who generally must perform the procedure. By contrast, a PA or NP often can handle the entire patient encounter on behalf of a primary care physician – by diagnosing the flu, for example, and prescribing the appropriate drugs.

This is an age of specialization in almost every field – from medicine to team sports, where we now have players who only rush the passer or only pitch the middle innings of a baseball game. It is unrealistic to believe that this trend will completely lose momentum, and even more unrealistic to believe that it will reverse itself. Generalist physicians will still have a key role to play in patient diagnosis and in the direction of patient care. But they will not be the dominant players controlling access to the health care system as advocates of health reform once believed.

Due to the growing presence of PAs and NPs, and due to the increasing number of medical graduates who have chosen to practice primary care in recent years, there will be a relative balance between the supply and demand for generalist doctors in the immediate future. The need will be greatest in rural areas that are traditionally underserved, inner city areas, and among immigrant populations. There will be plenty of work for primary care physicians and they certainly will not have to worry about unemployment or underemployment. But supply and demand for primary care physicians will be in a general state of equilibrium.

So, to paraphrase Bill Murray in *"Caddy Shack:"*

"We've got that going for us. Which is nice."

The Importance of Teamwork

Today's health care team is interdependent. While the physician remains the quarterback of the team, he or she needs the support of the other members to be fully efficient and to achieve personal and organizational goals. This is particularly true regarding nurses. When physicians list what motivates them to work with one hospital versus another, a good nursing staff is usually the second thing on the list. The first requirement is that the hospital be located close to the physician's office. So of the things over which a hospital has any control, a full, competent nursing staff is the number one perquisite for physicians.

Physicians are concerned that their patients receive appropriate, attentive care. Often, this boils down to a nurse being on the floor to monitor the patient, to answer questions, and to provide comfort. Life for doctors becomes more tedious, more complicated, and potentially more litigious when there are not enough nurses to see patients. They have to do more of the basic patient "rounding" themselves, the patients often feel neglected or angry, and they can be in a more legally confrontational frame of mind.

In addition to a full nursing staff, doctors like to see all- around efficiency in the hospital. This means that their patients are admitted quickly, that they have access to the appropriate diagnostic tests, and that test results come back in a timely manner. Efficiency often is undermined, however, when there are too few technologists on site to take x-rays, for example, or to process laboratory tests.

Insufficient allied professional staffing levels contribute to a feeling of tension and of constantly overtaxed resources that can be prevalent in many health care settings. It is one reason why health care sometimes presents a problematic work environment for doctors, which in turn drives some from the profession and causes others to warn young people away from it.

In this sense, the shortage of allied health professionals is helping to perpetuate the shortage of physicians. The result is a vicious cycle – a cycle that must be broken.

But how?

CHAPTER 12:
Where Do We Go From Here?

"You got to be careful if you don't know where you're going, because you might not get there." – Yogi Berra

The last chapter ended with a question – the main question we hope this book will raise among health professionals, political leaders and anyone else concerned about patient access to health care in America. The question is: How do we ensure that America will have the physicians it needs?

A second question the book poses – less directly, but perhaps more urgently for some readers – is whether or not becoming a physician is still worthwhile today. Should you as a young person set your sites on medical school? And, if so, what type of physician should you become?

We will address the second question first – mainly because it's easier to answer and we think the answer is more definite.

"I Want You Should Become a Doctor"

It's just about every mother's dream (Jewish mothers and otherwise) that their son or their daughter become a doctor. Not a jazz singer: a doctor. Is this still a worthy ambition in the American health care system as we have come to know it?

The short answer is, "of course." Medicine is still a great profession – the noblest profession of them all. There is a god-like power in being able to help or heal the sick – an incredible rush to be had in delivering a baby or in repairing or replacing a damaged heart. Medicine is a skill that transcends all borders and all divisions. Good physicians are welcomed everywhere.

This is truer today than it has ever been. Today's doctors have a much greater range of treatments and procedures at their command than has ever been the case in the past. This is made abundantly clear by the medical breakthroughs and miracles you read about almost daily – from the separation of conjoined twins to new discoveries in genetics.

Though they may not be on the pedestal that they once were, surveys show that physicians still lead all other professionals when it comes to public trust and respect. In polls, patients demonstrate that while they may have complaints about the health system as a whole, they are very satisfied with the performance of the individual physicians they see.

Moreover, at a time when job security in many professions is shaky, job security in medicine is extremely stable. We have already made the point that there is no such thing as an unemployed physician, and this book clearly demonstrates that the employment picture for doctors will be very positive for years to come. In addition, while it is true that many doctors have to work harder to maintain their earnings, incomes for physicians still are solidly upper middle class.

Medicine does exact its price, however, and anyone thinking about a medical career should approach the field with unclouded eyes. The requirements to "join the club" are steep – years of education and a great deal of expense are necessary before you can earn the right to be called a doctor. As we have discussed, the medical environment today sometimes resembles a minefield that has to be carefully negotiated. You are likely to be sued. Regulatory and reimbursement related paperwork will try your patience. After years of training and hands-on experience, you won't enjoy being second guessed by insurance company or government bureaucrats.

But if the science, the skill and the power of medicine thrill you – go for it. There are hassles and frustrations inherent to any profession, but the rewards offered by medicine are unique.

Having determined to enter medicine, what sort of physician should you become? Hundreds of young people have asked us this question over the years, and our response has always been the same. Choose the specialty you find the most intellectually and emotionally rewarding. Don't make your selection based on the projected job market for any particular field of medicine five, ten, or 15 years out. A good physician with a positive bedside manner who can lead a medical team will always find a welcome in the job market, regardless of his or her specialty. The challenges of medicine are daunting, so select a specialty that will give you the highest emotional and intellectual rewards in the long-term.

And good luck – we need you.

Where Do We Go From Here?

If the problem is simply that we need more physicians, then the answer appears to be equally simple – train more of them.

It will not be easy, however, to change the pattern of medical education and training in America. The first thing required is the political will to alter the established system. There is a great deal of public concern and political interest in our health care system, but the focus has always been on creating payment plans that allow greater access to health care. We haven't thought quite as much about *who will provide healthcare* should we devise a system that is more open to all.

The fact is, lines to get into the ER and wait times to see physicians will have to get even longer before the doctor shortage gets the political attention it deserves. That is unfortunate, because it will take quite a bit of time to increase the supply of physicians in America. First, money will have to be found to expand current medical schools and build more of them. While private grants and donations are used for this purpose, much of medical school education is paid for by the federal government and state governments. The federal deficit already is out of control, and many states facing budget shortfalls are cutting medical services, not budgeting for new training programs. Of course, in addition to educating more medical students, the number of medical residency programs will have to be expanded and the cap on federal spending on such programs will have to be lifted.

Should resources for facility expansion be found, the schools and training programs would need faculty. Medical faculty is increasingly hard to come by – we have noted already that many health professional training programs have to turn away qualified applicants because there are not enough teachers to go around. The schools also would need students. Historically, the number of applicants to medical schools has greatly exceeded the number of openings. However, as the cost of medical school and training reaches the upper regions of the stratosphere, and as youngsters are warned away from the profession, this may not always be the case.

Let us assume, however, that at some point the political will and the financial and human resources to train more physicians are found. It will take a minimum of seven to eight years from the moment a new medical school opens its doors before that school will have any impact on physician supply. When it comes to training physicians, we take our time and do the job right. The result is that no quick fix to our physician shortage problem is available.

Keeping What We Have

Until such time as we can train more physicians, we need to focus on keeping those we have, and on ensuring that medicine remains a profession attractive to young people.

A good first step would be streamlining or eliminating some of the onerous regulatory burdens doctors face. The coding and documenting requirements for physicians have simply gotten out of hand and must be simplified or eliminated where possible. Another positive step – one that many states are taking – is malpractice reform. We need to take those big, red bull's eyes off the backs of our physicians while ensuring reasonable redress for those patients with legitimate malpractice grievances.

The most intractable problem, however, is our current schizophrenic system of paying for health care. Doctors are put in an untenable position because everyone seems to want healthcare but no one seems to want to pay for it. The government looks to cut payments to physicians when it can, and private insurance companies follow suit. Since doctor bills usually are mostly paid by a third party, most patients don't sense the true cost of health care. It is going to be difficult to persuade older doctors to stay in medicine, or to attract young people to the field, unless they can see that society accepts a basic fact: that health care is worth paying for. The fight to justify and receive payment for their services is becoming too much for some physicians – to the point where they will are either quitting or accepting cash only.

Here we have hit upon the broad issue of health care reform – which is outside the scope of this book and more than we are willing or able to take on. Our only hope is that somewhere in this exhaustive debate the powers that be will factor in the vital element of physician supply.

The Few, the Proud

Physician supply is constrained in this country for one reason we would not wish to tamper with. You must be highly intelligent and highly motivated to become a medical doctor. The entire medical education and training establishment is set up to be exclusionary. You have to meet high standards to get into the system, and you have to maintain them to stay in. It is hard to conceive that at any point in time we would be overrun by people with the intellect and the temperament to be physicians. That is one reason why our system of medical education and training is considered to be the best in the world. Relaxing standards merely to increase physician supply would be a mistake and the proposition is not even on the table.

Even in the event that we are able to train more doctors – and we believe that this is imperative -- medicine will remain the exclusive domain of the most gifted and dedicated people America has to offer.

We wouldn't want it any other way.

***

SURVEYS

Following are the results of three surveys conducted by
The MHA Group:

2004 Survey of Physician
Appointment Wait Times

2005 Survey of Hospital
Physician Recruitment Trends

2005 Survey of Physician
Recruiting Incentives

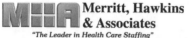

Merritt, Hawkins & Associates
"The Leader in Health Care Staffing"

Summary Report
2004 SURVEY OF PHYSICIAN APPOINTMENT WAIT TIMES

OVERVIEW

Merritt, Hawkins & Associates is a national physician search and consulting firm   specializing in the recruitment of physicians in all medical specialties.   Established in 1987, Merritt, Hawkins & Associates has conducted over 25,000 physician search assignments and has worked in all 50 states.

In order to better understand trends influencing the recruitment of physicians, Merritt, Hawkins & Associates conducts ongoing surveys on a wide range of health care staffing topics.   Previous surveys we have conducted have examined physician recruiting incentives, hospital physician recruiting practices, the practice patterns of older physicians, the practice preferences of final-year medical residents, and the average inpatient and outpatient revenue generated for hospitals by physicians in various medical specialties.

In recent years, Merritt, Hawkins & Associates has observed a sharp increase in the demand for medical specialists, which we attribute to a variety of factors.   These include an aging population, population growth, patient treatment preferences, expanding surgical, diagnostic, and pharmacological options, and the rise of payment plans that allow more direct patient access to specialists.   The growth in demand for physician services has been accompanied by a reduction in the supply of some specialists, due to shifting patterns of medical education, physician aging and retirement, evolving physician practice patterns, and changing physician demographics.

The result is that patient access to specialists has become increasingly problematic.   This is most directly observed in hospital emergency departments, where patients are routinely diverted due to a lack of medical specialists willing or available to treat emergency patients. Through our continuous professional contact with thousands of physicians, Merritt, Hawkins & Associates has observed that the length of time patients must wait for a physician appointment also appears to be lengthening.   In addition, a growing number of physicians appear to be unwilling or unable to schedule Medicaid patients.

The **2004 Survey of Physician Appointment Wait Times** was conducted to determine the average time new patients must wait before they can see a physician in a variety of large metropolitan markets.   The survey also examines the percentage of physicians willing or able to schedule Medicaid patients.   The survey is intended to gauge patient access to medical services and may be taken by health care professionals as one indicator of the current state of physician supply and demand in select markets   and in select medical specialties.

1

METHODOLOGY

During the months of February, March and April of 2004, research associates at Merritt, Hawkins & Associates called physician offices in 15 metropolitan areas with the purpose of scheduling a new patient appointment. The survey focused on four medical specialties: Cardiology, Dermatology, Obstetrics-Gynecology, and Orthopedic Surgery. Names of physicians were selected from Internet physician office listings at random, with an attempt to contact physician offices located in different parts of each metropolitan area.

Merritt, Hawkins & Associates selected a limited number of specialties in order to better focus available resources. The amount of time necessary to call physician offices, make contact with a receptionist, and schedule an appointment can be extensive. We determined to limit the number of specialties in order to increase the physician office sample size per specialty.

Merritt, Hawkins & Associates' research associates were tasked with contacting a minimum of 12 separate physician offices per specialty, per metropolitan area, and a maximum of 20 offices, with 20 being the preferred goal. Due to difficulties in reaching physician offices or to varying physician office scheduling policies, they were unable to contact 20 separate offices in all cases.

In each call, research associates asked to be told the first available time for a new patient appointment. Depending on the specialty at issue, they indicated a hypothetical, non-emergent reason for the appointment, as follows:

Cardiology   A heart check-up

Dermatology   A routine skin examine to detect possible carcinomas/melanomas

Orthopedic Surgery   Injury or pain in the knee

Obstetrics/Gynecology Routine "well woman" gynecological exam

Research associates also asked if the physician in question accepted Medicaid as a form of payment.

Merritt, Hawkins & Associates' goal was to replicate the experience of someone new to a community, with private insurance, seeking to schedule a non-emergent physician appointment through a generally accessible source, such as the Internet, the Yellow Pages, or a PPO physician directory. Phone research was conducted during an eleven week period. The results therefore are a "snapshot" of physician accessibility at a particular time and in a particular place. A change in timing or approach could yield different results.

Metropolitan service areas in which surveys were conducted:

Atlanta, Boston, Dallas, Denver, Detroit, Houston, Los Angeles, Miami, Minneapolis, New York, Philadelphia, Portland, San Diego, Seattle, Washington, D.C.

When survey was conducted:

February 1, 2004 - April 20, 2004

Medical specialties surveyed:

Cardiology, Dermatology, Obstetrics-Gynecology, Orthopedic Surgery

Number of surveys completed:

1,062

Total telephone calls required to complete 1,062 surveys:

Approximately 2,500

RESPONSES BY SPECIALTY

Cardiology

City	Total Responses	Shortest Time to Appt.	Longest Time to Appt.	Average Time to Appt.	Accept Medicaid? YES
Boston	18	7 days	120 days	37 days	11%
Philadelphia	20	1 day	136 days	27 days	80%
Portland	20	2 days	128 days	25 days	100%
Denver	20	2 days	128 days	23 days	20%
New York	20	3 days	26 days	22 days	0%
Miami	15	3 days	45 days	21 days	40%
Detroit	17	7 days	42 days	20 days	65%
San Diego	19	9 days	72 days	17 days	68%
Atlanta	20	3 days	28 days	17 days	80%
Minneapolis	20	2 days	105 days	15 days	80%
Los Angeles	18	1 day	23 days	14 days	22%
Washington, D.C.	16	Same day	23 days	12 days	100%
Houston	20	2 days	43 days	11 days	85%
Dallas	17	2 days	16 days	10 days	0%
Seattle	18	1 day	24 days	9 days	0%
Total:	**278**	**3.0 days**	**65.8 days**	**18.8 days**	**50%**

Dermatology

City	Total Responses	Shortest Time to Appt.	Longest Time to Appt.	Average Time to Appt.	Accept Medicaid? YES
Boston	18	7 days	120 days	50 days	17%
Minneapolis	19	9 days	231 days	43 days	100%
Dallas	14	10 days	70 days	34 days	0%
Philadelphia	20	6 days	140 days	33 days	15%
Portland	20	3 days	50 days	30 days	100%
Seattle	15	2 days	117 days	27 days	27%
Detroit	20	5 days	68 days	25 days	25%
Denver	20	Same day	60 days	21 days	20%
Atlanta	20	2 days	68 days	21 days	100%
Miami	14	1 day	55 days	17 days	71%
Washington, D.C.	15	Same day	32 days	15 days	87%
Los Angeles	16	Same day	36 days	14 days	50%
Houston	20	2 days	91 days	13 days	0%
San Diego	18	2 days	43 days	12 days	33%
New York	20	Same day	17 days	9 days	0%
Total:	**269**	**3.3 days**	**80.9 days**	**24.3 days**	**43%**

Obstetrics-Gynecology

City	Total Responses	Shortest Time to Appt.	Longest Time to Appt.	Average Time to Appt.	Accept Medicaid? YES
Boston	16	3 days	126 days	45 days	56%
Detroit	20	8 days	90 days	39 days	40%
San Diego	15	2 days	96 days	31 days	80%
Portland	20	1 day	79 days	30 days	100%
Philadelphia	17	8 days	72 days	28 days	24%
Seattle	17	1 day	153 days	26 days	70%
Atlanta	20	3 days	57 days	24 days	25%
Denver	20	1 day	33 days	23 days	25%
Minneapolis	15	6 days	61 days	20 days	80%
Houston	18	5 days	69 days	20 days	72%
Los Angeles	16	1 day	52 days	19 days	69%
Dallas	15	1 day	60 days	17 days	100%
New York	20	1 day	29 days	14 days	5%
Washington, D.C.	20	2 days	22 days	11 days	100%
Miami	12	3 days	12 days	10 days	50%
Total:	**261**	**3.0 days**	**65.1 days**	**23.3 days**	**60%**

Orthopedic Surgery

City	Total Responses	Shortest Time to Appt.	Longest Time to Appt.	Average Time to Appt.	Accept Medicaid? YES
Los Angeles	14	1 day	112 days	43 days	0%
Boston	16	1 day	60 days	24 days	88%
Denver	20	2 days	36 days	23 days	40%
Portland	20	Same day	26 days	19 days	100%
Minneapolis	14	7 days	93 days	19 days	79%
Philadelphia	16	4 days	76 days	18 days	25%
Detroit	18	5 days	48 days	18 days	22%
New York	20	2 days	39 days	16 days	10%
Houston	20	5 days	38 days	15 days	30%
San Diego	14	5 days	36 days	13 days	0%
Seattle	14	3 days	27 days	12 days	79%
Miami	14	7 days	21 days	11 days	14%
Dallas	14	2 days	18 days	10 days	43%
Washington, D.C.	20	1 day	25 days	8 days	20%
Atlanta	20	Same day	12 days	8 days	100%
Total:	**254**	**2.8 days**	**43.0 days**	**16.9 days**	**44%**

AVERAGE WAIT TIMES BY METROPOLITAN AREA

City	Cardiology	Dermatology	OB/GYN	Orthopedic Surgery
Atlanta	17 days	21 days	24 days	8 days
Boston	37 days	50 days	45 days	24 days
Dallas	10 days	34 days	17 days	10 days
Denver	23 days	21 days	23 days	23 days
Detroit	20 days	25 days	39 days	18 days
Houston	11 days	13 days	20 days	15 days
Los Angeles	14 days	14 days	19 days	43 days
Miami	21 days	17 days	10 days	11 days
Minneapolis	15 days	43 days	20 days	19 days
New York	22 days	9 days	14 days	16 days
Philadelphia	27 days	33 days	28 days	18 days
Portland	25 days	30 days	30 days	19 days
San Diego	17 days	12 days	31 days	13 days
Seattle	9 days	27 days	26 days	12 days
Washington, D.C.	12 days	15 days	11 days	8 days

MEDICAID ACCEPTANCE RATE BY METROPOLITAN AREA

City	Cardiology	Dermatology	OB/GYN	Orthopedic Surgery
Atlanta	80%	100%	25%	100%
Boston	11%	17%	56%	88%
Dallas	0%	0%	100%	39%
Denver	20%	20%	20%	40%
Detroit	65%	25%	40%	22%
Houston	85%	30%	72%	30%
Los Angeles	22%	50%	29%	14%
Miami	40%	71%	50%	14%
Minneapolis	80%	100%	83%	79%
New York	0%	0%	5%	10%
Philadelphia	80%	15%	24%	75%
Portland	100%	100%	100%	100%
San Diego	68%	33%	80%	0%
Seattle	0%	27%	70%	79%
Washington, D.C.	100%	87%	100%	46%

TRENDS AND OBSERVATIONS

Merritt, Hawkins & Associates' **2004 Survey of Physician Appointment Wait Times** is intended to present a "snapshot" of physician availability in four select medical specialties in a variety of metropolitan areas nationwide. In so far as it was possible, we attempted to duplicate the experience a person might have who sought to make a new patient appointment with a physician for a non-emergent medical problem.

This effort was necessarily subject to the varying appointment making policies of physician offices – vagaries that are not directly reflected in the core data above. For example, many physician offices employ answering machines that direct those seeking appointments to leave a message. In such instances, our research associates left a voice message as directed, requesting a follow-up call to schedule an appointment. In many cases, however, they were not able to reach the physician's office after two or more tries. In such cases, they no longer called the physician but moved on to other physician offices on their lists.

Merritt, Hawkins & Associates' research associates encountered other obstacles when seeking to obtain new patient appointment times. Some physician offices required verification of insurance before indicating when appointment times were available.

Timing also was an issue. In some cases, appointments "opened up" due to cancellations that occurred the day our research associates called. The core data above, therefore, only represent those instances in which our research associates were able to reach a physician's office and obtain a clear answer regarding the date of the first available new patient appointment.

The general anecdotal picture provided by our research associates is one in which many physician offices are hard to reach, so that scheduling an appointment can be difficult. They also reported that obtaining an answer to the question, "When is your first available appointment for a new patient?" is more problematic than it may first appear. Exceptions were noted, however, and in some cases physician offices were readily accessible and information was easy to obtain.

New Patient Wait Times by Specialty

The **2004 Survey of Physician Appointment Wait Times** is the first such survey Merritt, Hawkins & Associates has conducted, and therefore we cannot compare current wait times to any previous benchmark. In addition, as non-clinicians, we are unable to comment on the clinical effect these wait times may have on patients reporting non-emergent problems similar to the hypothetical ones stated by our research associates.

We can, however, make some inferences regarding the general availability of physicians based on the wait times reported for the four specialties at issue. In our experience in evaluating physician practices and in conducting hospital medical staff plans, a physician generally is considered busy if his or her practice is booked for new patient appointments two to three weeks in advance. In such cases, the recruitment of a new physician partner or associate may be warranted. It also is at this point that patients in the community begin to voice concerns about physician accessibility.

By this standard, average wait times indicated in the survey suggest that the majority of physician offices in most specialties are busy. In cardiology, average patient wait times were at or exceeded 14 days in 11 of the 15 metropolitan markets surveyed (73%). Cardiology wait times were at or exceeded 21 days in six of the 15 metropolitan markets surveyed (40%).

In dermatology, average patient wait times were at or exceeded 14 days in 12 of the 15 metropolitan markets surveyed (80%). Dermatology wait times were at or exceeded 21 days in 9 of the 15 metropolitan markets surveyed (60%).

In obstetrics-gynecology, average patient wait times were at or exceeded 14 days in 13 of the 15 metropolitan markets surveyed (87%). Obstetrics-gynecology wait times exceeded 21 days in 7 of the 15 metropolitan markets surveyed (47%).

In orthopedic surgery, patient wait times exceeded 14 days in 9 of the 15 metropolitan markets surveyed (60%). Orthopedic surgery wait times exceeded 21 days in 3 of the 15 metropolitan areas surveyed (20%). It is important to note that in calling orthopedic surgery offices our research associates reported having pain in the knee or in another joint, whereas in the other specialties they did not report having immediate pain.   Even when our research associates reported pain, however, average patient wait times extended to as long as 43 days in at least one market (Los Angeles).

Patient Wait Times At Or Exceeding 14 Day Wait Time Per Specialty

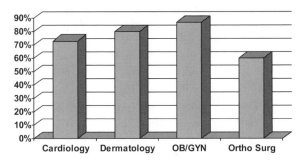

Patient Wait Times At Or Exceeding 21 Day Wait Time Per Specialty

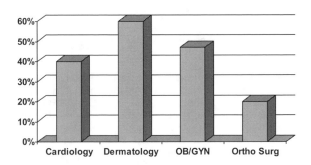

New Patient Wait Times By Market

Patient wait times in some of the 15 markets surveyed showed a consistent pattern in which wait times were relatively long or relatively short in most or all of the four specialties at issue.

Boston, for example, reported the longest average patient wait times in three of the four specialties surveyed, and it reported the second longest average wait times in the fourth specialty (orthopedic surgery.)   Though the Boston area supports a number of physician teaching hospitals that put new physicians into the work force every year, our experience in recruiting to the area indicates that Boston is having challenges in physician retention. A high managed care presence and rising malpractice rates are causing many physicians to leave the area and are making it increasingly difficult to attract physicians to Boston. This may account in part for the apparent difficulty in scheduling patient appointments there.

At the other end of the spectrum, average wait times reported for Washington, D.C. were consistently low. In three of the four specialty areas at issue, average patient wait times were 12 days or less, and only extended to an average of 14 days in dermatology. Washington, D.C. has the highest per capita ratio of physicians per population in the country, with 718 physicians per 100,000 people, as reported by the American Medical Association (Idaho, by contrast, has the lowest ratio; 178 physicians per 100,000 population.) This high physician-to-population ratio may explain the relative ease of scheduling a physician appointment in the D.C. area.

Highest & Lowest Average Wait Times In Days By Metro Market

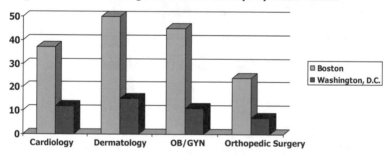

Other markets showed contrasts in wait times based on the specialty at issue. Los Angeles, for example, reported relatively moderate average wait times of 14 days in cardiology and dermatology, and 19 days in obstetrics-gynecology, but a relatively long average wait time of 43 days in orthopedic surgery, the longest average wait time for orthopedic surgery of any market surveyed.

Variations in wait times may be attributable to a variety of factors, including the net number of physicians per-population in a metropolitan area, demographic variations and disease incidence of the population, and prevalent health and lifestyle choices of the population.

It should be noted that all 15 metropolitan markets surveyed represent major population centers where physicians, specialists in particular, typically congregate. Most of these cities enjoy a higher ratio of physicians per population than many less populous areas, and a significantly higher ratio of physicians per population than many rural areas. Access to physician specialists in less populous areas could be expected to be more problematical than in the 15 metropolitan areas surveyed, though that would have to be confirmed by a separate survey.

Medicaid Rates of Acceptance

Medicaid acceptance rates also varied from one metropolitan area to the next, and variations among the four specialties were observed within the same metropolitan area.

In Dallas, for example, none of the cardiology or dermatology offices surveyed indicated that they accept Medicaid, while 100% of the obstetrics-gynecology offices surveyed indicated that they do accept Medicaid.   In Philadelphia, 80% of cardiology physician offices surveyed indicated that they do accept Medicaid, while 76% of obstetrician-gynecology offices indicated that they do not.

Some markets, by contrast, were more consistent.   In Portland, for example, all physician offices in all specialties reported that they accept Medicaid.   In New York, none of the cardiology or dermatology offices surveyed indicated that they accept Medicaid, and only 5% of obstetrics-gynecology offices and 10% of orthopedic surgery offices indicated that they accept Medicaid.

Highest & Lowest Medicaid Acceptance Rate By Metro Market

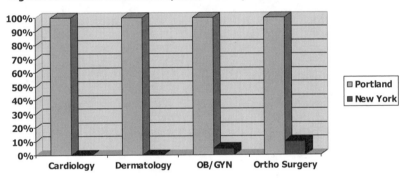

The rate at which physicians accept Medicaid can vary for a number of reasons.   In some cases, reimbursement rates provided by Medicaid to particular specialists may be below their cost of providing services.   If not actually below costs, Medicaid reimbursement often is relatively low compared to that offered by other payors, and busy physicians may have no economic incentive to see Medicaid patients.   In other cases, the process of billing for and receiving Medicaid payment can be problematic and some physicians choose to avoid it.

Medicaid patients comprise many of the patients who present to hospital emergency departments nationwide.   Often, lack of access to private practice physicians compels Medicaid patients to seek treatment in hospital emergency rooms.   The survey confirms that lack of access to physicians is a significant problem in some areas but not an impediment to physician access in others.

There is evidence, however, that the growing number of patients presenting to hospital emergency departments nationwide is being driven not by Medicaid patients or the uninsured, but by privately insured patients. An October, 2003 report by the Center for Studying Health System Change indicates that privately insured patients accounted for most of the 16% rise in hospital emergency department visits between 1996-97 and 2000-01. Many of these patients are not truly in need of emergency care, but they have found it difficult to see a private practice physician in the time frame that they are comfortable with, and so they seek physician care at a hospital emergency department. **The 2004 Survey of Physician Patient Wait Times** indicates that patient appointment times in some markets may be long enough to cause even insured patients to seek treatment at a hospital emergency department.

Merritt, Hawkins & Associates intends to conduct the Survey of Physician Patient Wait Times on a periodic basis to determine if any change in wait times is occurring over time. Information regarding additional surveys conducted by Merritt, Hawkins & Associates is included on the following page.

The MHA Group / Additional Surveys

Merritt, Hawkins & Associates is part of **The MHA Group**, a national organization of healthcare staffing firms. The MHA Group includes:

Merritt, Hawkins & Associates: Permanent physician & allied healthcare professional placement
Staff Care, Inc.: Locum tenens (temporary) physician staffing
Med Travelers: Temporary allied healthcare professional staffing
RN Demand: Temporary registered nurses
MTI Staffing: Temporary therapy professional staffing

Other surveys conducted by The MHA Group:

- Review Physician Recruitment Incentives
- Survey of Physicians 50 to 65 Years Old
- Physician Inpatient / Outpatient Revenue Survey
- OB/GYN Malpractice Survey
- Hospital Physician Recruitment Trends Survey
- Review of Temporary Healthcare Staffing Trends & Incentives
- Review of Temporary Healthcare Staffing Trends & Incentives (Mid-level providers)
- Review of Temporary CRNA Staffing Trends
- Review of Temporary Healthcare Staffing Trends in Psychiatry

For additional information about this survey or other surveys Merritt, Hawkins & Associates has conducted, please contact:

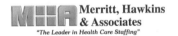

Merritt, Hawkins & Associates
"The Leader in Health Care Staffing"

www.merritthawkins.com
800-876-0500
5001 Statesman Drive
Irving, Texas 75063

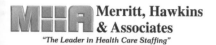
Merritt, Hawkins & Associates
"The Leader in Health Care Staffing"

SUMMARY REPORT
2005 Survey of Hospital Physician Recruitment Trends

Overview

Merritt, Hawkins & Associates (MHA) is a national physician search and consulting firm that periodically conducts surveys regarding a wide range of physician staffing issues. Prior surveys conducted by MHA have examined the types of recruiting incentives offered to physicians, the amount of revenue physicians generate for their affiliated hospitals, the practice patterns of older physicians, and the practice preferences of final-year medical residents.

This report summarizes the results of MHA's second survey of hospital recruiting trends and procedures. The survey is intended to provide benchmarking data regarding the percentage of hospitals currently recruiting physicians, types of physicians being recruited, and the methods hospitals are using to recruit physicians. The survey also indicates to what extent physician recruiting is a strategic priority for hospitals and the relative ease or difficulty hospitals are experiencing in recruiting various types of physicians.

The survey may prove useful to hospitals assessing their physician recruiting strategies, to medical staff planners interested in physician demand issues, and to physicians curious about hospital recruiting practices and trends.

Methodology

The 2005 Survey of Hospital Physician Recruitment Policies and Trends was mailed to 3,000 in-house hospital physician recruiters in 47 states in March, 2005. Names of in-house hospital physician recruiters were provided to MHA at random by a national health care database company.

By April 20, 2005, 312 completed surveys had been received, for a response rate of 10%. Survey results were tabulated over the following weeks and the Summary Report of results was completed in May, 2005. Merritt, Hawkins & Associates conducted a similar survey in 2002. The 2002 survey, however, was mailed to hospital chief executive officers, and not all of the questions asked in 2005 corresponded to questions asked in 2002. Though some of the responses from 2002 have been included in this report by way of comparison, the disparities in the two surveys should be considered by those seeking to track hospital physician recruiting trends over time.

2005 SURVEY OF HOSPITAL PHYSICIAN RECRUITING TRENDS

	Surveys mailed	Responses received	Response rate
2005	3,000	312	10%
2002	3,000	280	9%

1

QUESTIONS ASKED AND RESPONSES RECEIVED (all numbers rounded to the nearest full digit)

1. **What is the size of your hospital?**

	2005	2002
100 beds or less	39%	60%
101-200 beds	29%	22%
201 beds or more	32%	18%

2. **Is your hospital currently recruiting physicians?**

	2005		2002	
	Yes	**No**	**Yes**	**No**
100 beds or less	75%	25%	78%	22%
101-200 beds	95%	5%	99%	1%
201 beds or more	98%	2%	96%	4%
Overall Total:	**88%**	**12%**	**85%**	**15%**

3. **If yes, what types of physicians are you now recruiting? (of 277 hospitals currently recruiting)**

	100 beds or less	**101-200 beds**	**201 beds or more**	**2005 Total**	**2002 Total**
Allergist	-	2%	8%	3%	>1%
Anesthesiologist	9%	15%	24%	15%	20%
Cardiologist	9%	35%	48%	29%	>1%
Dermatologist	5%	12%	16%	10%	7%
Endocrinologist	3%	12%	26%	13%	6%
Family Practitioner	42%	37%	47%	43%	45%
Gastroenterologist	6%	20%	35%	19%	14%
General Surgeon	27%	19%	38%	30%	27%
Geriatrician	-	2%	10%	4%	1%
Hematologist/Oncologist	3%	14%	28%	14%	11%
Hospitalist	12%	31%	43%	28%	10%
Infectious Disease	-	5%	7%	4%	5%
Internal Medicine	25%	44%	54%	40%	32%
Maternal/Fetal Medicine	-	2%	10%	4%	>1%
Neurologist	6%	25%	31%	20%	12%
Neurosurgeon	2%	8%	35%	14%	1%
Nuclear Medicine	-	-	2%	1%	1%
OB/GYN	16%	29%	32%	25%	21%
Occupational Medicine	-	6%	7%	4%	1%
Ophthalmologist	-	2%	4%	2%	1%

	100 beds or less	101-200 beds	201 beds or more	2005 Total	2002 Total
Orthopedic Surgeon	27%	53%	42%	40%	33%
Pathologist	1%	2%	6%	3%	4%
Pediatrician	9%	14%	17%	13%	14%
Pediatric Subspecialties	-	-	15%	5%	2%
Psychiatrist	7%	13%	50%	23%	14%
Plastic Surgeon	2%	6%	13%	8%	1%
Pulmonologist	6%	15%	24%	14%	9%
Radiologist	8%	18%	24%	16%	14%
Rheumatologist	3%	7%	14%	8%	8%
Urgent Care	3%	1%	7%	4%	1%
Urologist	9%	21%	27%	19%	15%
Vascular Surgeon	4%	15%	19%	12%	6%

4. **Based on your most recent recruitment efforts, please rate how difficult the following specialties are to recruit:**

	Not particularly difficult (1-2)		Somewhat difficult (3)		Very difficult (4-5)	
	2005	2002	2005	2002	2005	2002
Allergist	30%	-	40%	-	30%	
Anesthesiologist	25%	14%	33%	37%	42%	49%
Cardiologist	8%	9%	15%	44%	77%	47%
Dermatologist	N/A	25%	N/A	34%	N/A	41%
Endocrinologist	11%	-	27%	-	62%	-
Family Practitioner	58%	68%	32%	19%	10%	13%
Gastroenterologist	8%	18%	17%	46%	75%	36%
General Surgeon	20%	20%	35%	55%	45%	25%
Geriatricians	35%	-	30%	-	35%	-
Hematologist/Oncologist	13%	11%	30%	48%	58%	41%
Hospitalists	37%	-	40%	-	13%	-
Infectious Disease	40%	-	27%	-	33%	-
Internal Medicine	18%	42%	45%	45%	37%	13%
Maternal/Fetal Medicine	21%	-	12%	-	67%	-
Neurologists	13%	-	24%	-	63%	-
Neurosurgeons	10%	N/A	7%	N/A	83%	N/A
Nuclear Medicine	22%	-	48%	-	30%	-
OB/GYN	33%	17%	31%	46%	36%	37%
Occupational Medicine	44%	-	41%	-	15%	-
Ophthalmologist	40%	-	31%	-	29%	-
Orthopedic Surgeon	11%	8%	11%	34%	78%	58%
Pathologist	51%	-	32%	-	17%	-
Pediatrician	57%	44%	26%	45%	17%	11%
Pediatric Subspecialties	20%	12%	19%	45%	61%	43%

	Not particularly difficult (1-2)		Somewhat difficult (3)		Very difficult (4-5)	
	2005	2002	2005	2002	2005	2002
Psychiatrist	20%	-	20%	-	60%	-
Plastic Surgeon	26%	-	25%	-	49%	-
Pulmonologist	13%	-	23%	-	74%	-
Radiologist	12%	8%	15%	-	73%	63%
Rheumatologist	16%	10%	27%	44%	57%	46%
Urgent Care	68%	-	16%	-	16%	-
Urologist	11%	7%	15%	42%	74%	52%
Vascular Surgeon	17%	-	24%	-	79%	-

5. Where does physician recruitment stand as a priority for your hospital?

A top priority	62%
Important, but not a top priority	30%
Somewhat important	8%
Relatively unimportant compared to other issues	0%

6. What methods do you currently use to recruit physicians?

	100 beds or less		101-200 beds		201 beds or more	
	2005	2002	2005	2002	2005	2002
Advertising in medical journals	31%	40%	52%	40%	71%	20%
Advertising on job web sites	33%	53%	55%	28%	73%	19%
Direct Mail to physicians	24%	%	52%	%	52%	%
Contingent physician recruiting firms	70%	54%	79%	27%	76%	19%
Retained physician recruiting firms	41%	53%	56%	25%	43%	22%
Exhibiting at physician conventions	15%	49%	17%	22%	31%	29%
Networking with residency programs	53%	58%	57%	23%	69%	19%
Networking with medical staff/ community	61%	56%	79%	26%	81%	18%

7. Rate the effectiveness of any of the recruiting methods you use:

	Least effective (1-2)	Somewhat effective (3)	Most effective (4-5)
Advertising in medical journals	55%	29%	16%
Advertising on job web sites	30%	32%	48%
Direct Mail to physicians	41%	38%	21%
Contingent physician recruiting firms	35%	26%	39%
Retained physician recruiting firms	22%	33%	45%
Exhibiting at physician conventions	63%	23%	14%
Networking with residency programs	25%	30%	45%
Networking with medical staff/ community	14%	23%	63%

8. Do you currently pay physician specialists to cover your hospital's emergency department?

Yes	37%
No	63%

9. In the last 12 months, has physician recruitment at your facility become:

More difficult and time consuming	24%
Less difficult and time consuming	3%
Stayed the same	69%
N/A	4%

10. Consider your hospital's working relationship with its physician staff. In the last 12 months, have physician/hospital relations at your facility:

Improved	40%
Become worse	14%
Stayed the same	46%

11. Please rate the physician recruiting challenges facing your hospital:

	Least difficult(1-2)	Somewhat difficult (3)	Most difficult (4-5)
Geographic location to our facility	33%	17%	50%
Ability to offer competitive incentives	46%	25%	29%
Overall shortage of physicians	23%	42%	35%
Finding physicians who fit our facility's parameters	18%	27%	55%
Meeting requirements of the physician's spouse	29%	28%	43%
Exhibiting at physician conventions	63%	23%	14%

12. Has your hospital changed or revised physician recruiting contracts in light of the indictment of a national health system for alleged violations of physician recruiting laws?

Yes	29%
No	71%

13. **Is your hospital concerned by the fact that Stark II limits the financial assistance hospitals can provide to established groups seeking to recruit another physician?**

Yes	54%
No	42%
Not aware of Stark II recruiting limitation	4%

14. **The association of American Medical Colleges is holding a seminar to consider physician supply. Do you believe the U.S. medical education system needs to train more physicians?**

Yes	92%
No	8%

TRENDS AND OBSERVATIONS

Merritt, Hawkins & Associates' 2005 Survey of Hospital Physician Recruiting Trends reveals a variety of physician recruitment patterns and policies currently prevalent in hospitals of various sizes located nationwide.

The great majority of in-house hospital physician recruiters surveyed -- 88% -- indicated that their facilities are actively recruiting physicians. The percentage is higher for larger hospitals. Ninety-five percent of in-house recruiters at hospitals of 101-200 beds indicate their facilities are recruiting physicians, as do 98% of recruiters at hospitals of 201 or more beds. Several types of physicians are being recruited with particular frequency. More hospital recruiters (43%) indicated their facilities are actively involved in searches for family practitioners than for any other kind of medical specialist. Other frequently recruited specialists include general internists, who the survey indicates are being recruited by 40% of hospitals, orthopedic surgeons, also being recruited by 40% of hospitals, general surgeons, who are being recruited by 30% of hospitals surveyed, and cardiologists, who are being recruited by 29% of hospitals surveyed.

Types of physicians being recruiting varies by hospital size. Fifty-percent of hospitals of 201 beds or more report recruiting psychiatrists, compared to 13% of hospitals of 101-200 beds and 7% of hospitals of 100 beds or less. For hospitals of 201 beds or more, psychiatry trails only general internal medicine as the most frequently recruited specialty. Larger facilities are more likely to include psychiatric wards than smaller ones, and the high rate of psychiatry recruitment in these facilities reflects what Merritt, Hawkins & Associates views as the increasing demand for a wide range of mental health services nationwide.

There are a variety of other medical specialties more commonly available at larger hospitals than smaller hospitals, and these are being recruited with greater frequency at larger facilities than smaller ones. These specialties include dermatology, endocrinology, gerontology, hematology/oncology, hospitalists, maternal/fetal medicine specialists, neurologists, neurosurgeons, pediatric sub-specialists, plastic surgeons, rheumatologists, urologists, and vascular surgeons.

Among smaller hospitals of 101 beds or less, family practitioners, general surgeons, and orthopedic surgeons are the most sought after types of specialists, the survey indicates, followed by general internists. At least 25% of recruiters at smaller hospitals indicated their facilities are recruiting these types of physicians. By contrast, no more than 16% of recruiters at smaller hospitals indicated they were recruiting any other type of physician. In many instances, smaller hospitals are located in rural areas where shortages of primary care physicians persist. These hospitals also often focus on basic services, such as general surgery, obstetrics, and orthopedic surgery and rarely offer surgical subspecialties such as neurosurgery, plastic surgery and other services.

Which physicians are the most difficult to recruit?

The survey indicates that while family practitioners and general internists are being recruited more frequently than other types of doctors, they are not the most difficult types of physician to recruit.

Recruiters were asked to rate which types of doctors are the most difficult to recruit on a scale of 1-5, with 5 being the highest degree of difficulty. Eighty-three percent of recruiters surveyed indicated that neurosurgeons rated a 4 or a 5 on the scale, suggesting that neurosurgeons are more difficult to recruit today than any other type of physician.

A variety of other specialists also were rated as very difficult to recruit, including cardiologists, gastroenterologists, orthopedic surgeons, pulmonologists, radiologists, urologists, and vascular surgeons. At least 73% of recruiters surveyed rated these specialties as a 4 or a 5 on the scale of difficulty. Increases in demand for these services and a relatively limited supply combine to make recruitment in these areas difficult.

By contrast, two types of primary care physicians, family practitioners and pediatricians, were rated as relatively easy to recruit. Fifty-eight percent of those surveyed rated family practitioners as a 1 or a 2 of the scale of difficulty, while 57% rated pediatricians as a 1 or a 2. In primary care (defined by Merritt, Hawkins & Associates as family practice, pediatrics, and internal medicine), only general internists were consistently rated as somewhat difficult or very difficult to recruit. This may be explained to some extent by the supply situation in primary care. For much of the 1990's, the number of primary care residents increased dramatically, helping to keep supply and demand in relative balance for the near term. We anticipate this will change in coming years as fewer medical graduates currently are training in some areas of primary care -- family practice in particular. The delayed effect of this drop in supply is likely to be felt in the next four to five years.

Recruiting methods and challenges

Hospital physician recruiters surveyed employ a variety of methods to recruit doctors. The methods recruiters use vary somewhat by size of hospital, but in some cases patterns are consistent. At least 40% of recruiters in hospitals of all sizes indicate that they use contingent search firms, networking with the hospital's medical staff/community, networking with residency programs, and retained physician recruitment firms to recruit physicians.

In some cases, methods hospital use to recruit physicians do vary by size of hospital. For example, 71% of recruiters in hospitals of 201 beds or more indicated that they use advertising in medical journals as a recruitment method, compared to only 31% of recruiters in hospitals of 100 beds or less. In addition, 73% of recruiters in hospitals of 201 beds or more indicated they use job web sites to recruit, compared to 33% of recruiters in hospitals of 100 beds or less.

The frequency by which certain recruiting methods are used may be tied to their relative cost. Contingent recruitment firms and networking are both widely used by hospitals of all sizes. No payment is required to contingent firms unless a placement is made and networking also may entail activities such as meeting with physicians that generate few costs. Smaller hospitals in particular appear to favor those recruiting methods that require relatively little costs, while larger facilities appear to embrace a wider variety of recruiting methods regardless of costs.

Recruiters at hospitals of all sizes appear to agree that networking with the facility's medical staff is the most effective method of physician recruitment. Over 60% of recruiters surveyed indicated that this type of networking was the most effective. Forty-five percent or more of those surveyed also rated advertising on job web sites, retained physician recruiters, and networking with residency programs to be most effective.

The most difficult challenge in physician recruitment as rated by those surveyed is finding physicians who fit the facility's parameters. This challenge was rated more difficult than the facility's geographic location, its ability to offer competitive incentives, the physician shortage, or the challenge of meeting the requirements of the physician's spouse. This suggests that regardless of national trends in physician supply and regardless of economic considerations, physician recruiting remains essentially a matchmaking process in which the basic challenge is to find the right physician for a particular facility.

Federal regulations and the physician shortage

The majority of hospital physician recruiters surveyed (71%) indicate that the high profile indictment of a for-profit facility for alleged physician recruitment violations has not caused their hospitals to revise their physician recruiting contracts. However, over one quarter of those surveyed (29%) indicate that their hospitals have changed their physician contracts in light of the indictment. This suggests that a significant number of facilities have concerns regarding the types of incentives they are offering to recruit doctors or the recruitment and retention methods their facilities are employing.

In addition, the majority of recruiters surveyed (54%) are concerned about Stark II regulations limiting the ability of hospitals to offer financial assistance to established medical groups seeking to recruit physicians. Combined, these responses reflect the widespread effect that recent federal activity is having on the physician recruitment market.

The survey also suggests that the majority of hospital physician recruiters would like to see steps taken to address the physician shortage. Ninety-two percent of those surveyed indicated that they believe the U.S. medical education system needs to train more physicians.

For additional information about this and other Merritt, Hawkins & Associates' surveys, please contact:

Merritt, Hawkins & Associates
"The Leader in Health Care Staffing"
800-876-0500
www.merritthawkins.com

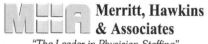
Merritt, Hawkins
& Associates
"The Leader in Physician Staffing"

SUMMARY REPORT
2005 Review of Physician Recruitment Incentives

OVERVIEW

Merritt, Hawkins & Associates is a national health care search and consulting firm specializing in the recruitment of physicians in all medical specialties and advanced practice allied professionals. Established in 1987, Merritt, Hawkins & Associates has conducted over 25,000 physician search assignments and has worked in all 50 states.

This report marks Merritt, Hawkins & Associates' twelfth annual review of the physician search and consulting assignments we conduct on behalf of our clients.

The 2005 Review is based on the combined 2,687 physician search and consulting assignments Merritt, Hawkins & Associates represented from April 1, 2004 to March 31, 2005.

The intent of the Review is to quantify financial and other recruitment incentives offered by our clients to physician candidates during the course of a 12-month period. The range of incentives detailed in the Review may be used as one benchmark for evaluating which recruitment incentives are customary and competitive in today's physician recruiting market. In addition, the Review, which is based on a national sample of physician search assignments, provides an indication of which medical specialties are currently in the greatest demand.

All of the following numbers are rounded to the nearest full digit.

Total Number of Physician Search Assignments Reviewed

2004/05	**2003/04**	**2002/03**	**2001/02**
2,687	2,594	2,405	2,220

Medical Settings of Physician Search Assignments

	2004/05	**2003/04**	**2002/03**	**2001/02**
Group	1,290 (48%)	1,089 (42%)	938 (39%)	910 (41%)
Partnership	242 (9%)	571 (22%)	529 (22%)	488 (22%)
Solo	492 (18%)	519 (20%)	433 (18%)	365 (16%)
Hospital	510 (19%)	285 (11%)	313 (13%)	310 (14%)
Association	48 (2%)	78 (3%)	96 (4%)	67 (3%)
HMO	0 (0%)	0 (0%)	0 (0%)	15 (1%)
Other	105 (4%)	52 (2%)	96 (4%)	65 (3%)

49 States Where Search Assignments Were Conducted

AK, AL, AR, AZ, CA, CO, CT, DE, FL, GA, HI, IA, ID, IL, IN, KS, KY, LA, MA, MD, ME, MI, MO, MN, MS, MT, NC, ND, NE, NH, NJ, NM, NY, NV, OH, OK, OR, PA, SC, SD, TN, TX, UT, VA, VT, WA, WI, WV, WY

Number of Searches by Community Size

	2004/05	2003/04	2002/03	2001/02
0-25,000	806 (30%)	622 (24%)	625 (26%)	621 (28%)
25,001-100,000	860 (32%)	960 (37%)	866 (36%)	777 (35%)
100,001+	1,021 (38%)	1,012 (39%)	914 (38%)	822 (37%)

Top Fifteen Searches By Medical Specialty (total of 1,743 searches)

	2004/05	2003/04	2002/03	2001/02
Cardiology	231	181	188	226
Radiology	218	202	230	252
Orthopedic Surgery	210	210	191	172
Internal Medicine	188	124	113	152
Family Practice	166	165	122	135
General Surgery	116	112	84	90
Gastroenterology	94	105	69	102
OB/GYN	83	103	110	112
Psychiatry	80	54	59	49
Anesthesiology	64	98	134	131
Hospitalist	62	82	55	41
Neurosurgery	62	52	58	48
Urology	59	94	56	61
Neurology	56	60	44	30
Otolaryngology	54	52	42	32

Comparison of Top 5 Searches: 2004/05 to 2003/04

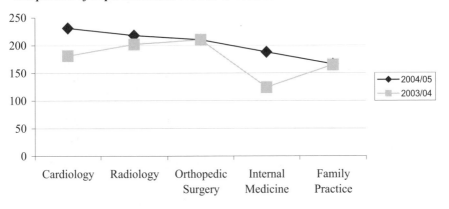

Other Specialty Recruitment Assignments (944 total searches)

Allergy
Cardiovascular Surgery
Critical Care/Pediatrics
Dermatology
Geriatrics
Hand Surgery
Infectious Disease
Neonatology
Occupational Medicine
Orthopedic Foot & Ankle Surgery
Pain Management
Pediatric/Cardiology
Pediatric/Intensivist
Pediatric/Orthopedic Surgery
Pediatric Urology
Physiatry
Reproductive Endocrinology
Trauma Surgery

Bariatric Surgery
Child Psychiatry
Critical Care/Pulmonology
Endocrinology
Gynecology
Hematology/Oncology
Maternal/Fetal Medicine
Neurological Surgery
Ophthalmology
Orthopedic Spine Surgery
Pathology
Pediatric Emergency Medicine
Pediatric/Nephrology
Pediatric/Radiology
Perinatology
Plastic Surgery
Radiation Oncology
Urgent Care

Cardiothoracic Surgery
Colon/Rectal Surgery
CRNA
Endovascular Surgery
Gynecology/Oncology
Hospitalist
Nephrology
Neuroradiology
Oral Maxillofacial Surgery
Orthopedic Trauma Surgery
Pediatric/Anesthesiology
Pediatric/Endocrinology
Pediatric/Ophthalmology
Pediatric/Surgery
Pharmacy
Podiatry
Rheumatology
Vascular Surgery

Income Offered to Top 15 Recruited Specialties

	Low	Average	High
Cardiology			
2004/05	$234,000	$320,000	$525,000
2003/04	$230,000	$292,000	$500,000
2002/03	$230,000	$280,000	$475,000
2001/02	$220,000	$273,000	$500,000
Radiology			
2004/05	$250,000	$355,000	$500,000
2003/04	$240,000	$336,000	$450,000
2002/03	$230,000	$317,000	$500,000
2001/02	$240,000	$286,000	$600,000
Orthopedic Surgery			
2004/05	$250,000	$361,000	$650,000
2003/04	$240,000	$330,000	$500,000
2002/03	$230,000	$315,000	$450,000
2001/02	$220,000	$295,000	$450,000
Internal Medicine			
2004/05	$130,000	$161,000	$210,000
2003/04	$125,000	$152,000	$200,000
2002/03	$125,000	$150,000	$200,000
2001/02	$120,000	$148,000	$180,000

	Low	Average	High
Family Practice			
2004/05	$125,000	$150,000	$200,000
2003/04	$120,000	$146,000	$195,000
2002/03	$120,000	$146,000	$190,000
2001/02	$110,000	$144,000	$195,000
General Surgery			
2004/05	$220,000	$255,000	$310,000
2003/04	$210,000	$248,000	$300,000
2002/03	$200,000	$242,000	$275,000
2001/02	$185,000	$221,000	$280,000
Gastroenterology			
2004/05	$230,000	$298,000	$340,000
2003/04	$210,000	$250,000	$325,000
2002/03	$200,000	$240,000	$325,000
2001/02	$190,000	$226,000	$350,000
OB/GYN			
2004/05	$200,000	$247,000	$320,000
2003/04	$185,000	$242,000	$325,000
2002/03	$190,000	$237,000	$325,000
2001/02	$180,000	$219,000	$325,000
Psychiatry			
2004/05	$140,000	$176,000	$250,000
2003/04	$130,000	$164,000	$260,000
2002/03	$130,000	$162,000	$250,000
2001/02	$120,000	$153,000	$240,000
Anesthesiology			
2004/05	$240,000	$303,000	$340,000
2003/04	$220,000	$300,000	$325,000
2002/03	$225,000	$290,000	$325,000
2001/02	$200,000	$278,000	$325,000
Hospitalist			
2004/05	$150,000	$171,000	$210,000
2003/04	$140,000	$162,000	$200,000
2002/03	$135,000	$155,000	$180,000
2001/02	$130,000	$149,000	$170,000
Neurosurgery			
2004/05	$350,000	$424,000	$575,000
2003/04	$350,000	$420,000	$550,000
2002/03	$300,000	$390,000	$550,000
2001/02	$300,000	$370,000	$545,000

	Low	Average	High
Urology			
2004/05	$250,000	$329,000	$340,000
2003/04	$220,000	$294,000	$325,000
2002/03	$210,000	$277,000	$325,000
2001/02	$200,000	$245,000	$325,000
Neurology			
2004/05	$155,000	$209,000	$230,000
2003/04	$145,000	$191,000	$220,000
2002/03	$150,000	$180,000	$215,000
2001/02	$150,000	$170,000	$210,000
Otolaryngology			
2004/05	$235,000	$304,000	$350,000
2003/04	$230,000	$278,000	$350,000
2002/03	$225,000	$270,000	$375,000
2001/02	$215,000	$255,000	$300,000

Average Income Offers by Geographic Region

Geographic regions are defined as follows:

Northeast	**Southeast**	**Midwest**	**West**
Maine	Virginia	Texas	New Mexico
New Hampshire	West Virginia	Oklahoma	Arizona
Vermont	Tennessee	Missouri	Colorado
Rhode Island	Kentucky	Illinois	Nevada
Massachusetts	North Carolina	Indiana	Wyoming
Pennsylvania	South Carolina	Ohio	Montana
Connecticut	Florida	Michigan	Idaho
New Jersey	Georgia	Wisconsin	California
New York	Alabama	Minnesota	Utah
Delaware	Mississippi	Kansas	Oregon
Maryland	Louisiana	Nebraska	Washington
	Arkansas	Iowa	Hawaii
		North Dakota	
		South Dakota	

(Not included: Alaska)

Average Income Offers by Geographic Region

	Northeast	Southeast	Midwest	West
Cardiology	$310,000	$330,000	$330,000	$312,000
Radiology	$340,000	$360,000	$362,000	$310,000
Orthopedic Surgery	$351,000	$370,000	$370,000	$345,000
Internal Medicine	$155,000	$164,000	$164,000	$164,000
Family Practice	$145,000	$152,000	$151,000	$144,000
General Surgery	$245,000	$260,000	$262,000	$248,000
Gastroenterology	$290,000	$300,000	$302,000	$285,000
OB/GYN	$245,000	$250,000	$250,000	$240,000
Psychiatry	$170,000	$178,000	$178,000	$172,000
Anesthesiology	$295,000	$310,000	$305,000	$294,000
Hospitalist	$165,000	$175,000	$174,000	$165,000
Neurosurgery	$170,000	$178,000	$178,000	$172,000
Urology	$320,000	$334,000	$335,000	$320,000
Neurology	$202,000	$212,000	$215,000	$200,000
Otolaryngology	$280,000	$295,000	$290,000	$280,000

Type of Incentive Offered

	Salary	Salary w/ Bonus	Income Guarantee
2004/05	269 (10%)	1,478 (55%)	940 (35%)
2003/04	233 (9%)	1,296 (50%)	1,065 (41%)
2002/03	289 (12%)	1,202 (50%)	914 (38%)
2001/02	355 (16%)	1,110 (50%)	755 (34%)

Type of Guarantee (of 940 Searches Offering Guarantees)

	Net Collections Guarantee	Gross Collections Guarantee
2004/05	827 (88%)	113 (12%)
2003/04	916 (86%)	149 (14%)
2002/03	749 (82%)	165 (18%)
2001/02	589 (78%)	166 (22%)

Term of Guarantee (of 940 Searches Offering Guarantees)

	1 Year	2 Year	3 Year	Other
2004/05	708 (75%)	220 (23%)	8 (1%)	4 (1%)
2003/04	852 (80%)	203 (19%)	10 (1%)	0 (0%)
2002/03	713 (78%)	192 (21%)	9 (1%)	0 (0%)
2001/02	568 (75%)	176 (23%)	6 (1%)	5 (2%)

Searches Offering "Forgiveness" of Guarantee (of 940 Searches Offering Guarantees)

	Forgiveness	**No Forgiveness**
2004/05	884 (94%)	56 (6%)
2003/04	1,012 (95%)	53 (5%)
2002/03	859 (94%)	55 (6%)
2001/02	672 (89%)	83 (11%)

Time Period of Forgiveness (of 884 Searches Offering Forgiveness)

	1 Year	**2 Year**	**3 Year**	**Other / N/A**
2004/05	38 (4%)	547 (58%)	303 (32%)	52 (6%)
2003/04	30 (3%)	516 (51%)	405 (40%)	61 (6%)
2002/03	26 (3%)	310 (36%)	429 (50%)	94 (11%)
2001/02	5 (1%)	229 (34%)	319 (47%)	119 (18%)

Paying Relocation

	Yes	**No**
2004/05	2,677 (99%)	10 (1%)
2003/04	2,578 (99%)	16 (1%)
2002/03	2,379 (99%)	26 (1%)
2001/02	2,181 (98%)	39 (2%)

Amount of Relocation Allowance

	Low	**Average**	**High**
2004/05	$3,500	$8,850	$20,000
2003/04	$2,000	$9,250	$22,000
2002/03	$2,000	$9,000	$20,000
2001/02	$2,000	$9,066	$20,000

Signing Bonus Offered

	Yes	**No**
2004/05	1,236 (46%)	1,451 (54%)
2003/04	1,290 (50%)	1,304 (50%)
2002/03	866 (36%)	1,539 (64%)
2001/02	777 (35%)	1,443 (65%)

Amount of Bonus

	Low	Average	High
2004/05	$5,000	$14,030	$50,000
2003/04	$5,000	$15,500	$45,000
2002/03	$4,500	$15,000	$50,000
2001/02	$5,000	$14,270	$50,000

Paying Continuing Medical Education

	Yes	No
2004/05	2,498 (93%)	189 (7%)
2003/04	2,412 (93%)	182 (7%)
2002/03	2,212 (92%)	193 (8%)
2001/02	2,022 (92%)	198 (8%)

Amount of CME

	Low	Average	High
2004/05	$1,000	$3,350	$15,000
2003/04	$1,500	$3,250	$10,000
2002/03	$1,500	$3,100	$10,000
2001/02	$1,000	$3,097	$10,000

Paying Additional Benefits

	2004/05	2003/04	2002/03	2001/02
Health Insurance	92%	96%	96%	93%
Malpractice	93%	90%	91%	94%
Retirement	72%	70%	72%	74%
Disability	74%	70%	72%	75%
Educational Loan Forgiveness	14%	16%	12%	11%

TRENDS AND OBSERVATIONS

Merritt, Hawkins & Associates' annual **Review of Physician Recruiting Incentives** tracks data derived from the national physician recruitment assignments that the firm conducts over the 12 month period ranging from April 1 of one year to March 31 of the next.

The types of physician recruiting assignments Merritt, Hawkins & Associates conducts, and the incentives its client offer to recruit physicians, may be of interest to health care administrators, physician recruiters and others who follow developments in the areas of physician staffing, physician compensation and physician supply and demand.

The 2005 Review reflects a variety of ongoing and emerging physician recruiting trends. In the 12 month period covered by the 2005 Review, Merritt, Hawkins & Associates conducted search assignments in all 50 states, with the exception of Rhode Island. This suggests that at least some hospitals, medical groups and other health care organizations in all parts of the country have found physician recruitment to be a challenge and require outside assistance.

From 1987, when Merritt, Hawkins & Associates was established, to 2000, the plurality of searches the firm conducted were in communities of 25,000 people or less. Since 2000, however, the plurality of searches we have conducted have been in communities of 100,001 or more. For example, in the 12 month period covered by the 2005 Review, Merritt, Hawkins & Associates conducted 30% of its searches in communities of 25,000 or less, 32% of its searches in communities of 25,001 to 100,000, and 38% of its searches in communities of 100,001 or more.

The locations of our recruiting assignments indicate that physician recruiting challenges are no longer regionalized but are prevalent in communities of all sizes in all areas of the country. Indeed, Merritt, Hawkins & Associates now conducts recruiting assignments on behalf of health care facilities in highly desirable coastal and mountain resort areas; facilities which in the past did not require physician recruiting assistance due to their favorable locations. In addition, we now conduct physician recruiting assignments on behalf of some of the most recognizable health care institutions in the world, institutions which in previous years had little trouble attracting physician candidates on their own.

The steady growth in the number of search assignments we conduct, which has doubled from 1,352 in 1995/96 to 2,687 in 2004/05, further reflects the growing demand for physicians and the diminishing supply of candidates nationally.

The Top 15

Merritt, Hawkins & Associates' top 15 search assignments in the 12 month period covered by the annual Review indicates to some extent which medical specialties are in the greatest demand. More specifically, these assignments reflect which specialties are both in demand and difficult to recruit. According to Merritt, Hawkins & Associates' 2005 Survey of Hospital Physician Recruiting Trends, more hospitals are actively engaged in recruiting family physicians than any other type of physician. However, cardiology, not family practice, was our number one search assignment in 2004/05. This apparent dichotomy is due to the fact that family practitioners are generally not as difficult to recruit as cardiologists. Some facilities today can recruit family physicians on their own but may require the assistance of an outside firm to recruit cardiologists and other specialists.

While cardiology, radiology and orthopedic surgery have topped the list of our most frequently conducted search assignments for the last five years, two areas of primary care, internal medicine and family practice showed continued or renewed prominence in the 2005 Review. The number of internal medicine search assignments Merritt, Hawkins & Associates conducted increased from 124 in 2003/04 to 188 in 2004/05, a growth rate of 51%. This growth can be attributed in part to the enhanced need for internists among a growing population of elderly patients. In addition, some facilities that are unable to recruit a sufficient number of internal medicine sub-specialists turn to general internists to address their needs.

The number of family practice search assignments Merritt, Hawkins & Associates conducted dropped from 694 in 1996/97 to 122 in 2002/04. However, in 2003/04, the number of family practice searches we conducted increased to 165. This increase held steady at 166 family practice search assignments in 2004/05. These increases indicate a steady resurgence in two areas of primary care recruitment as hospitals and other health care providers seek to meet the needs of changing demographics and/or maintain patient referral networks. However, a third area of primary care (pediatrics) dropped out of our top 15 search assignments for the first time since we began compiling data.

Also noteworthy among the top 15 searches is the growth in psychiatry. The number of psychiatry searches Merritt, Hawkins & Associates conducted increased from 54 in 2003/04 to 80 in 2004/05, a growth rate of 48%. In last year's Review, we anticipated this growth due to both a growing demand for behavioral health services and a diminishing supply of psychiatrists. Psychiatrists are, on average, one of the oldest medical specialists and the number of medical students choosing to specialize in psychiatry is declining. A growing number of facilities, many of them state funded mental health facilities or correctional facilities, are unable to recruit the psychiatrists they need and are reliant on temporary (i.e., *locum tenens)* practitioners to fill gaps in their staffs. We project that psychiatrists will become increasingly difficult to recruit and that the need for additional psychiatrists will become acute in the next five to 10 years.

Neurosurgery is another specialty that is becoming increasingly difficult to recruit. Neurosurgery was among Merritt, Hawkins & Associates' top 15 most recruited specialties in 2004/05, the first time it has been on the list. The supply of neurosurgeons has traditionally been limited, while population growth is fueling demand. Even those hospitals with a sufficient number of neurosurgeons are finding it difficult to persuade these specialists to cover their emergency departments, causing a growing number of patient transfers from one facility to another.

By contrast, demand for both obstetrician/gynecologists and anesthesiologists showed declines in this year's Review. Falling birthrates in many areas may explain the dwindling demand for OB/GYNs, while a number of facilities addressed their needs in anesthesiology in the previous four to five years, during which time the volume of search assignments Merritt, Hawkins & Associates conducted in anesthesiology sharply increased. In addition, anesthesiology is one of the few medical specialties where a significant amount of care can be provided by non-physicians, and in many cases health care organizations are recruiting certified registered nurse anesthetists (CRNAs) in lieu of anesthesiologists.

Income Offers Reflect Growing Demand

The 2005 Review indicates that the base income offered to recruit physicians continues to spike as the demand for medical services outpaces the supply of available physicians.

The average income offered to recruit cardiologists increased from $292,000 last year to $320,000 this year, the average offer to orthopedic surgeons increased from $330,000 last year to $361,000 this year, and the average offer to radiologists increased from $336,000 last year to $355,000 this year. By contrast, in the 1998/99 Review, the average income offer to cardiologists was $206,000, the average offer to orthopedic surgeons was $245,000 and the average offer to radiologists was $197,000.

Other areas showing significant increases over last year include gastroenterology, up from $250,000 last year to $298,000 this year, otolaryngology, up from $278,000 last year to $304,000 this year, urology, up from $294,000 last year to $329,000 this year and internal medicine, up from $152,000 last year to $161,000 this year.

The 2005 Review marks the second year we have tracked income offers by geographic region. As in last year's Review, the 2005 Review indicates that average income offers are generally higher in the Southeast and Midwest than they are in the Northeast and the West. The variations generally are not pronounced, however, because the physician recruitment market is national in scope and offers generally have to be competitive on a national rather than a regional basis.

In addition to the base financial offer, other incentives are used to recruit physicians. Relocation is a standard incentive and was paid for in virtually all of the assignments Merritt, Hawkins & Associates conducted in 2004/05. The average relocation allowance provided by our clients dipped slightly from $9,250 in 2003/04 to $8,550 this year. Signing bonuses were offered in 46% of search assignments conducted in 2004/05, down from 50% last year but up from 36% and 35% the two previous years. The average signing bonus offered by Merritt, Hawkins & Associates' clients was $14,030 in 2004/05, compared to $15,500 last year.

Continuing medical education is a standard incentive, offered in 93% of searches conducted in 2000/05, with no change from last year. The average CME allowance offered grew marginally from $3,250 in 20003/04 to $3,350 in 2004/05. Health insurance, malpractice insurance, retirement and disability are increasingly common incentives, each of them offered in 80% or more of the searches Merritt, Hawkins & Associates conducted in 2004/05

Summary

Merritt, Hawkins & Associates' 2005 Review of Physician Recruiting Incentives underscores the fact that the demand for physicians is national and that communities in all areas of the country require some outside assistance in physician recruitment. Demand for cardiologists, radiologists and orthopedic surgeons remains high, while demand for psychiatrists and neurosurgeons is spiking. The 2005 Review shows a steady increase in demand in two areas of primary care (internal medicine and family practice) while demand in obstetrics/gynecology and anesthesiology appears to be diminishing. Financial incentives reflect the growing demand for physicians and are up significantly for many specialists. The 2005 Review indicates that financial incentives offered to recruit physicians are generally higher in the Southeast and Midwest than they are in the Northeast and the Northwest and that certain incentives such as relocation and continuing medical education are standard in the industry.

The MHA Group / Additional Surveys

Merritt, Hawkins & Associates is part of **The MHA Group**, a national organization of healthcare staffing firms. The MHA Group includes:

Merritt, Hawkins & Associates: Permanent physician and allied healthcare professional placement
Staff Care, Inc.: Locum tenens (temporary) physician staffing
Med Travelers: Temporary allied healthcare professional staffing
MTI Staffing: Temporary therapy professional staffing
RN Demand: Temporary registered nurses staffing

Other surveys conducted by The MHA Group:

- Survey of Physician Appointment Wait Times
- Survey of Physicians 50 to 65 Years Old
- Physician Inpatient / Outpatient Revenue Survey
- Survey of Final Year Medical Residents
- Hospital Physician Recruitment Trends Survey
- Review of Temporary Healthcare Staffing Trends & Incentives
- Review of Temporary Healthcare Staffing Trends & Incentives (Mid-level Providers)
- Review of Temporary CRNA Staffing Trends
- Review of Temporary Healthcare Staffing Trends in Psychiatry

Books written by MHA Group executives:
Will the Last Physician in America Please Turn Off the Lights? A Look at America's Looming Physician Shortage
For additional information about this survey or other information generated by The MHA Group, please contact:

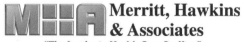

Merritt, Hawkins & Associates
"The Leader in Health Care Staffing"

Corporate Headquarters (800) 876-0500
www.merritthawkins.com

ABOUT THE MHA GROUP

Established in 1987, The MHA Group consists of five distinct staffing and consulting companies, including:

Merritt, Hawkins & Associates, Permanent Physician Search and Consulting

Staff Care, Inc., Temporary (Locum Tenens) Physician Staffing

Med Travelers, Temporary Allied Health Care Professional Staffing

MTI Staffing, Temporary Therapy Professional Staffing

RNDemand, Temporary Nurse Staffing

Together, The MHA Group of companies employs some 750 people in four national and regional offices and is the endorsed health care staffing provider of over 20 state hospital associations. The MHA Group is a subsidiary of AMN Healthcare, the nation's largest nurse staffing company. AMN Healthcare/The MHA Group is the largest healthcare staffing company in the United States.

For additional information about The MHA Group, please contact:

The MHA Group
5001 Statesman Drive
Irving, Texas 75063
800-876-0500
469-524-1400
www.mhagroup.com